Dinky's Health & Homeopathic

'Patrick Holford is one of the leading lights in nutritional medicine today. He has brought together new research and facts from the world's most respected nutritional scientists. It makes riveting reading – after the first page I was hooked. This book is a must for anyone who wants to become and remain healthy in these challenging times.'
HAZEL COURTENEY, *Sunday Times*

'There have been dramatic changes over the past decade in our views about healthcare and Patrick Holford has been right at the forefront of many of these changes, particularly with our revised appreciation of nutrition.

The road to bad medicine and bad health is built on the foundation of dogma. It is refreshing to have this dogma subjected to fresh examination. I commend this book to you on the basis that it is well researched and written with substantial backing of references from reliable scientific and medical journals. It is certainly a book well worth reading.'
DR JOHN MARKS, Life Fellow and former Director of Medical Studies, University of Cambridge

'*100% Health* is an excellent book. It is essential reading for the health-conscious and deserves a long success.'
EMANUEL CHERASKIN, Professor of Medicine and Dentistry, School of Medicine, University of Alabama

'This is an important book which deserves to influence orthodox medical thinking, and is both informative and up-to-date on health and nutrition issues for the lay reader.'
DEREK BRYCE-SMITH, Emeritus Professor of Chemistry, University of Reading

'Fascinating and inspiring. This is do-it-yourself health at its best.'
SHEENA MILLER, Editor of *Here's Health*

100%
HEALTH

The drug free guide to feeling better, living
longer and staying free from disease

PATRICK HOLFORD

PIATKUS

*The real act of discovery consists not in finding
new lands, but in seeing with new eyes*

MARCEL PROUST

First published in 1998 by
Judy Piatkus (Publishers) Ltd
5 Windmill Street, London W1P 1HF

Reprinted 1998

**The moral right of the author
has been asserted**

*A catalogue record for this book is available
from the British Library*

ISBN 0–7499–1813–6 Hbk
ISBN 0–7499–1968–X Pbk

Illustrations by Jonathan Phillips and Christopher Quayle
Designed by Paul Saunders

Typeset by Phoenix Photosetting, Chatham, Kent
Printed and bound in Great Britain by Biddles Ltd,, Guildford, Surrey

CONTENTS

Acknowledgements

With thanks to Bernard Gesch, Dr Jeffrey Bland, Professor Derek Bryce-Smith, Dr Fritjof Capra, Dr Emanuel Cheraskin, Professor Michael Crawford, Dr Stephen Davies, Dr Abram Hoffer, Oscar Ichazo, Dr John Lee, Kate Neil, Dr Richard Passwater, Dr Linus Pauling, Dr Carl Pfeiffer, Dr Alex Schauss, Dr Stephen Schoenthaler, Dr Evans Shute, Michael Walleczek and Dr Roger Williams for their contributions to this book and to humanity.

Guide to abbreviations and measures

1 gram (g) = 1000 milligrams (mg) = 1,000,000 micrograms (mcg or µg).
Most vitamins are measured in milligrams or micrograms. Vitamins A, D, and E are also measured in International Units (ius), a measurement designed to standardise the various forms of these vitamins that have different potenicies.

1mcg of retinol (mcg RE) = 3.3ius of vitamin A
1mcg RE of betacarotene = 6mcg of betacarotene
100ius of vitamin D = 2.5mcg
100ius of vitamin E = 67mg

1 pound (lb) = 16 ounces (oz)   2.2lb = 1 kilogram (kg)
1 pint = 0.6 litres   1.76 pints = 1 litre
In this book calories means kilocalories (kcals)

References and further sources of information

Hundreds of references from respected scientific literature have been used in writing this book. Details of specific studies referred to are listed on pp. 203–9. Other supporting research for statements made is available from the Lamberts Library at the Institute for Optimum Nutrition (ION) (see p. 210), whose members are free to visit and study there. ION also offers information services, including literature search and library search facilities, for those readers who want to access scientific literature on specific subjects. On p. 202 you will find a list of the best books to read, linked to each chapter, to enable you to dig deeper into the topics covered.

This book is about a revolution in healthcare – not just an update on advances in the treatment of modern diseases, but a radical rethink on the whole concept of health and disease, its causes and cures. Reading this book will change your way of looking at health. From this new viewpoint, different questions arise. The answers to those questions define the direction of medicine and healthcare in both the present and the future, and create a new way of living that can take you towards your full potential for health and vitality. Given the threats of future disease epidemics, escalating healthcare costs and ever-increasing stress, this book is an essential survival guide for the twenty-first century. It is a handbook for the health-conscious who want to live longer, feel better and stay free from disease.

PART 1

QUANTUM HEALTH

The significant problems we have created . . .
cannot be solved at the same level of thinking we
were at when we created them.

ALBERT EINSTEIN

ONE

A New Way of Looking

Few of us realise how much of what we think and see is shaped by the culture we are born into. If you were born in the 1700s the world was undoubtedly flat. Those who thought otherwise, despite having extensive evidence to prove it, were considered heretics and lunatics. In fact, it took two hundred years for the 'flat-earthers' to concede defeat and for people to accept that the world was round.

Right now the same shift is taking place in our understanding of health. Much of today's medicine and the way we consider our health is based on the theories of the physicist Sir Isaac Newton and his seventeenth- and eighteenth-century contemporaries. They saw the world, and the human body, as a machine made out of parts. To understand health, they believed, you just imagined each part and then put all the parts together to get the whole picture. Each part could be broken down and examined to find out how it worked. This kind of thinking led to hospitals with departments for each body system, the concept of transplants and surgical removal of parts that didn't work or weren't found to have a function – from your appendix to your tonsils.

The concept of germs causing disease, proved by Louis Pasteur in the nineteenth century, added the idea that disease was caused by some outside agent that needed to be eradicated usually by drugs or surgery. And so we entered the era of a 'drug for a bug' or a 'pill for an ill'. While this approach has produced some positive results, the concept of 'combat medicine' is failing to provide much-needed breakthroughs of most of the ill health we face today.

Consider some of the major diseases of modern times. What's on offer for them? Cancer treatment involves chopping it out, drugging it out or burning it out with radiation. For heart disease the options include bypassing the blocked artery, and taking drugs to relax the artery or thin the blood – all very 'mechanical' in concept. For arthritis, there are two kinds of drugs: non-steroidal anti-inflammatory drugs, like aspirin, and steroid drugs, like cortisone. Both kill the pain. But both speed up the progression of the arthritis. The same is true for many drug treatments and surgical procedures.

A single course of antibiotics increases a child's risk of ear infection by five times. Oestrogen HRT (hormone replacement therapy), taken over a decade, doubles a woman's risk of breast cancer. Even over-the-counter painkillers increase the risk of headaches, while decongestant cold cures increase the risk of strokes if used frequently.

Not only are side-effects a major problem, but the results are far from encouraging. Take breast cancer, for example. Currently, one in 12 women develops breast cancer in the USA, and one in 8 in the UK, and the numbers are rising. In truth, breast cancer is occurring more frequently and earlier in women's lives than a decade ago. By 2017 the prediction is that a woman's risk of developing cancer in her life is over 50 per cent, and a man's over 65 per cent. We are losing the cancer war, not winning.

Currently, more than half the population suffer from some chronic health problem, and 38 per cent of men and 47 per cent of women are constantly on prescribed medication.[1] The annual cost of the National Health Service is £40 billion – that's £700 per person per year.

There is one treatment that has consistently brought reductions in death rates. That's no treatment. An analysis of mortality rates from around the world shows rapid and significant declines when doctors go on strike. A month-long strike in Israel in 1973 halved the number of deaths, while a seven-week strike in Los Angeles in 1976, resulted in an 18 per cent reduction in deaths. 'It may be a coincidence but it is a fact,' said a spokesman for the

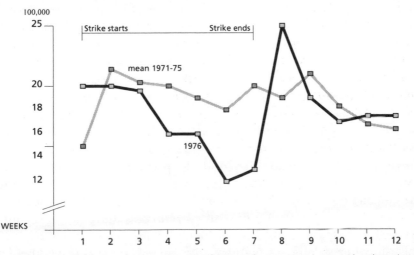

In 1976, doctors in Los Angeles went on strike for 6 weeks to protest increased malpractice insurance premiums. The death rate swiftly decreased below the year's average until the 7th week when the strike ended – initially death rate rose sharply surpassing the year's average until the 9-10th week when the death rate dropped to its yearly average.

Fig. 1   Death rates during doctors' strike

National Morticians Association. What's more, in the strikes analysed, mortality rates tend to return to normal when the strikes are over. One explanation for this could be the number of deaths from medical operations or from drug reactions. Non-steroidal anti-inflammatory drugs, first popularised as an alternative to dangerous steroid drugs, is now a $9.5 billion industry – $5 billion for the drug and $4.5 billion for treating the side-effects. Thousands of people die from the side-effects of these drugs alone. Whatever the cause of this phenomenon, perhaps it's time to question the old ideas upon which twentieth-century medicine has been based.

These are old ideas based on old ways of thinking that picture an invader (a bug, tumour or blockage) and a defender armed with an arsenal of scalpels, lasers and chemical weaponry. Unfortunately, the medical arms race still continues today. Yet too often the costs outweigh the benefits. What's more, few, if any, diseases are caused by a deficiency of drugs or surgery, so isn't it illogical that they should provide the cure? Isn't there something better on offer?

Any physicist will tell you that Newton is old hat. His ideas were useful to a point, but Einstein's ideas have taken us much further. But what was Einstein saying, and how does this relate to you and your health?

$$E = mc^2$$

Instead of viewing life (and disease) as a battle, Einstein believed that everything was not only interconnected but made of the same stuff, which he called 'energy'. He said that what we perceive as matter (m), that solid stuff like your body, is only energy (E) in motion (c). It's like the movies. A film is made of an image, then a space, then an image, then a space. But if you roll the film fast enough all you see is a moving image, not the space. If you look at your arm under a microscope you will see that it's made out of cells with spaces in between. If you look at a cell under a microscope it's made of protein, fat and a lot of water. These substances are made of smaller units that we call atoms, with space in between. The atoms are made of smaller units called electrons, protons and neutrons, with space in between. These electrons, protons and neutrons are made of even smaller particles called quarks, once again with space in between. In fact, if quarks were real matter, the entire matter of the human body would fit on to a pin head! The rest is empty space.

What Einstein was saying was that everything is the same energy, including the empty space, and that when energy 'condenses' we call it matter. This may all seem a bit abstract, but new ideas are. That's what makes them new.

In the old way of thinking, cancer is an 'invader' that has to be destroyed. We don't ask so much how it got there as how to get rid of it. In the new way of thinking we see all cells in the body as being, or containing, energy. Normally the energy is directed towards the health of the body. What, then, happens in a cancer cell? The evidence today points to the idea that cancer cells stop 'talking' to other cells and working for the good of the whole, and instead isolate themselves and become selfish. They enlarge and multiply, develop their own blood supply to get what they need, and start to take over the body like a megalomaniac.

What are the conditions that trigger a cell to stop communicating with other cells and working together? This idea of 'connectedness' is inherent in new concepts of health. Instead of just looking at the parts, modern approaches give equal importance to the 'relationship' or pattern of organisation of the parts. For example, instead of just looking for a cause of lung cancer, such as smoking, and a cure, such as vitamin C, we now understand that part of the risk for cancer is determined by one's total exposure to oxidants – generated from hundreds of sources such as sunlight, pollution, radiation, fried food, poor diet and smoking – versus one's total intake of hundreds of different kinds of anti-oxidants – including vitamins A, C and E found in food. If a person takes in too many oxidants in relation to their intake of antioxidants this can disrupt the way body cells behave in relation to each other, sometimes triggering cancer.

Another concept that came from modern physics is that the 'energy' in a system jumps from one level to another. In other words, things change in steps. Ice becomes water, water becomes steam. Our health doesn't gradually decline, day by day. One day you're well, the next day you're ill. One moment you're happy, the next moment you're depressed. Each step or stage is called a 'quanta', hence quantum physics and quantum health. If you put enough energy into a system it will jump to a higher level. If the system loses energy it will drop to a lower level. So the right diet, exercise and frame of mind increase available energy, while the wrong diet, lack of exercise and a negative frame of mind dissipate energy.

This idea of gaining and losing energy is like a cost-benefit equation. Drugs, surgery and radiation all cost the patient a lot of energy. So in these cases the potential 'cure' is itself increasing future risk of disease. There is a danger here in going round and round in circles. You give a drug to cure one disease, and create another. You take a drug to counteract the side-effects of another drug, and so on. Many medical scientists are beginning to question whether the costs of drugs such as antibiotics, synthetic hormones and anti-inflammatories really do outweigh the benefits.

Complex Adaptive Systems

Instead of viewing the body like a machine, medicine is finally beginning to look at human beings as complex adaptive systems, more like a self-organising jungle than a complicated computer. Rather than trying to 'control' a person's health by playing God with hi-tech medicine, there's a new way of looking at health that considers a human being as a whole, with an interconnected mind, body and spirit that is designed to adapt to health if the circumstances are right.

Of course, we are each born different and inherit a different level of resilience or adaptive capacity. So, in this new model, our health is a result of the interaction between our inherited adaptive capacity (our genes) and our circumstances or environment. If our environment is sufficiently hostile (bad diet, pollution, viruses, toxins, allergies etc.) we exceed our ability to adapt and get sick.

So, going back to cancer, we know that the risk is higher if you smoke, regularly drink alcohol, eat meat, take certain drugs and hormones, are exposed to exhaust fumes and other pollutants and are highly stressed, to name a few. The risks are, on the other hand, lower if you have a high intake of certain vegetables, fibre, antioxidant vitamins such as betacarotene, vitamin C and E, and live in a clean environment. Evidence shows that, when the pluses significantly outweigh the minuses, health can be improved. In other words, you can experience a quantum leap to better health.

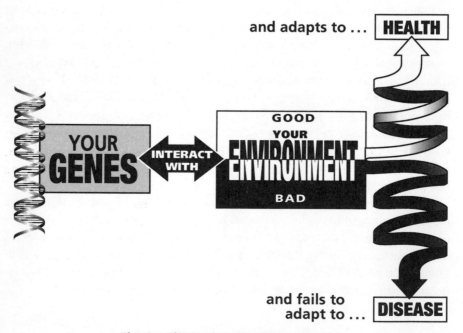

Fig. 2   The path to health or disease

TWO

THE DRUG DILEMMA

According to Dr Emanuel Cheraskin former Professor of Medicine, at the University of Alabama Medical School, 'healthcare today is the fastest-growing failing business'. While costs are escalating, health is decreasing. In the past twenty years the annual number of drug prescriptions in the UK has almost doubled, from 282 million in 1975 to 473 million in 1995. That's more than seven prescriptions per person per year!

While doctors swear to abide by the Hippocratic Oath, the main principles of which are 'First do no harm' and 'Assist nature', their behaviour more often resembles the principle 'First prescribe a drug, alien to the body's chemistry'. Dr Stephen Davies, founding editor of the *Journal of Nutritional Medicine*, calls this 'pharmacodoxic medicine'. It's not orthodoxy, since orthodox medicine is based on the principles of Hippocrates, but pharmacodoxy, in which the fundamental principle becomes 'First prescribe a pharmaceutical drug'. With tens of thousands of deaths brought about worldwide each year by the medical prescription of pharmaceutical drugs, this approach to medicine is hardly in line with the principle of first doing no harm and clearly has nothing to do with assisting nature.

Caught between the patient's desire for instant relief of pain, and the pharmaceutical industry's persuasive and profitable marketing of 'magic bullets', too much of modern medicine has become reliant on drugs. Most of these add to the burden of man-made toxins we are each exposed to, with consequent costs to the patient in terms of side-effects. Do these costs outweigh the benefits? Let's consider the five major types of drugs prescribed.

Painkillers

These account for 80 million prescriptions a year in the UK, which is a small proportion of the total annual consumption of painkillers, valued at £577 million or roughly £10 per person, most of which are bought over the counter. Paracetamol-based painkillers are notoriously toxic to the liver, and land 30,000 people in the UK in hospital each year.[2] According to Professor Sir David Carter of Edinburgh University, one in 10 liver transplants is due to the damage caused by paracetamol overdose.[3] Painkillers containing sali-cylic acid, such as aspirin, are gastrointestinal irritants[4] and adversely increase the permeability of the gut wall, leading to digestive problems, inflammation and allergies. Long-term use of painkillers is also associated with 'chronic daily headache'. According to consultant neurologist Dr Simon Ellis, painkillers should never be taken more than one day in four, or seven days a month.

Decongestant Drugs

These are found in over-the-counter cold cures and nose sprays and are thought to increase the risk of healthy people having a stroke. Medical researchers at the University of Pennsylvania Medical Center identified eight relatively healthy young stroke victims who had none of the usual risk factors, although seven had used decongestants on a long-term basis.[5] The researchers think that these drugs, which constrict blood vessels to dry up a cold or hay fever, may affect blood vessels elsewhere in the body, particularly in people who have migraines or Raynaud's disease, and whose blood vessels are therefore already constricted.

Anti-inflammatory Drugs

These fall into two categories: hormone-based derivatives of cortisone, and non-steroidal anti-inflammatories (NSAIDS). The former create a dependency so that the body reduces its own natural production of cortisone. Sudden withdrawal can be fatal. Long-term use is highly undesirable and associated with symptoms including facial swelling, unwelcome fatty deposits, muscle wasting, slow wound healing and increased risk of infection.[6] NSAIDS account for more drug-related deaths than any other category of pharmaceutical drugs, usually as a consequence of internal bleeding brought on by these drugs irritating the gut wall. Both these types of drug speed up the progression of arthritis.[7]

Antibiotics

These account for over 50 million annual prescriptions in the UK, roughly one per person per year. Not only are they intestinal irritants, wiping out the healthy intestinal bacteria that can take over three months to be restored, but their widespread use is leading to the development of drug-resistant strains of life-threatening bacteria from tuberculosis to gonorrhoea and staphylococcal infections, responsible for some sore throats. The US National Institute of Health estimate that, by the year 2000, a total of 50,000 tons of antibiotics will be used every year throughout the world on humans, animals and plants. Their use also increases the risk of repeat infections.

Antidepressants and Tranquillisers

These account for 3.6 million prescriptions a year in the UK and are very much on the increase. New drugs like Prozac, which accounts for $2.9 billion in annual sales worldwide, are being freely prescribed to children and adults alike at the slightest hint of depression. According to psychiatrist Dr David Richman, 10–25 per cent of people experience each of the following ten most common of the drug's forty-five known side-effects:

- nausea
- nervousness
- insomnia
- headache
- tremors
- anxiety
- drowsiness
- dry mouth
- excessive sweating
- diarrhoea

In spite of this, Prozac is considered one of the safest antidepressants. Dr Abram Hoffer, former Psychiatric Research Director for the Province of Saskatchewan in Canada, says that 'tranquillisers never cure mental illness because they only replace one psychosis with another'.

Synthetic Hormones

These have been given to billions of women, in the form of the birth control pill and hormone replacement therapy (HRT) at the menopause, without any real knowledge of the long-term effects. The short-term effects are bad enough – reflected in the fact that 6 in every 7 women stop HRT within one year of starting. The long-term effects range from increased risk of breast cancer to blood clots, weight gain and gynaecological problems. Even more concerning is the accumulating evidence that points to over-exposure to harmful oestrogenic chemicals (found mainly in plastics and pesticides) as

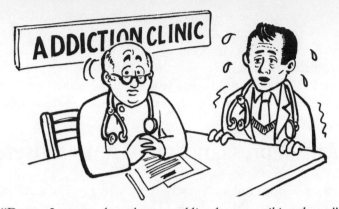

"Doctor, I seem to have become addicted to prescribing drugs."

a major contributor to the rapid decline in human fertility and abnormal sexual development in infants.

As the American Chemical Society registers its 10 millionth chemical, 18,000 of which the average person is exposed to each day; as the pharmaceutical industry records another year of growth exceeding 11.6 per cent, with a global annual turnover in excess of £178 billion; as the health records of the world's most affluent countries record increasing rates of ill health, visits to the doctor and hospital admissions, we have to wonder whether modern medicine is barking up the wrong tree.

THREE

THE GENETIC MYTH

The big buzz word in medicine is genetics. Ever since the discovery that a protein molecule, DNA, found in every cell of the body, contains genes which offer a set of instructions to determine how the body behaves, scientists have been scrambling to decipher the instructions and find ways to alter them for our apparent benefit.

Some of the first successes and disasters in genetic engineering have been restricted to plants and simple organisms. In 1989 a Japanese company started selling a form of tryptophan, an amino acid used in certain nutritional supplements, that had been produced by a new process involving genetic engineering. The resultant tryptophan was the cheapest on the market and soon found its way into supplements, but instead of nourishing people it made them sick. Twenty-seven people died and over 1000 were permanently disabled. To this day exactly what went wrong is still unknown.[8]

Genetically modified foods now include tomatoes, soya and maize. However, as much as half of supermarket foods are the product of some sort of genetic engineering. You are probably already eating them unknowingly. The purpose for genetically modifying soya was to make it resistant to herbicides. In other words, genetically modified soya is sprayed with herbicides that kill all weeds but not the plant, increasing the yield. We, the consumers, eat the herbicide residues and genetically modified soya, adding to our chemical load, while the agrochemical company Monsanto (which owns both the patent for the new strain of soya and the herbicide to which it is resistant) profits – and we are told that this technological advance is for the benefit of humanity! Monsanto, the fourth largest chemical company in the USA, claims that 'agricultural biotechnology' is needed to maintain the global population without harming the environment, and is spending millions of pounds in the UK alone to woo the public into accepting their genetically modified food.

Genetic Disease

Genetic defects play a major role in certain diseases such as cystic fibrosis, Down's syndrome, homocystinuria and other less common conditions. This list is, however, being lengthened to include almost every known degenerative condition, including cancer and heart disease – or so the newspapers report. The impression created is that each gene corresponds to a character trait or disease tendency which programs the individual for a certain behaviour or disease. It follows then, that hi-tech science is decoding the genes that give a propensity for a disease, so that some time in the future you too, like the tomato, can avoid disease by having your genes modified.

This linear, mechanistic description of genetics is not only completely inaccurate, it generates powerlessness and complacency. 'Well, if it's genetic there's not much I can do about it, is there? I'm programed to be fat, have asthma and die, like my parents, in my seventies.'

It's Not All in the Genes

In the case of genetics, truth is stranger and more complex than fiction. According to scientist Fritjof Capra, author of *The Web of Life*,

> While biologists know the precise structure of a few genes, they know very little of the ways in which genes communicate and cooperate in the development of an organism. In other words, they know the alphabet of the genetic code but have almost no idea of its syntax. It is now apparent that most of the DNA – perhaps as much as ninety-five per cent – may be used for integrative activities about which biologists are likely to remain ignorant as long as they adhere to mechanistic models.

Instead of one gene containing the instructions for one trait, a person's genetic make-up seems to be the result of highly complex interactions between the codes of numerous genes and the person's internal chemical environment. What's more, whether the instructions of any given gene are turned on or off depends again on the person's internal chemical environment. Instead of there being only one possible genetic programing of an individual, there are thousands if not millions of possible genetic expressions, determined more by the chemical environment of the individual than by their inherited genes. As medical biochemist Dr Jeffrey Bland says, 'Those codes, and the expression of the individual's genes, are modifiable. The person you are right now is the result of the uncontrolled experiment called "your life" in which you have been bathing your genes with experience to give rise to the outcome of that experiment. If you don't like the result of the experiment that makes up your life thus far, you can change it at any moment, whether you are 15 or 75 or 90.'

Consider the story of a former nurse called Mavis.[9] In her mid-sixties she suffered from severe asthma and frequent pneumonia and was going into hospital about twice a year. She was given antibiotics to clear her lung infections, but with each bout her lung function was gradually deteriorating. Mavis seemed to be losing ground and, faced with a bleak, short future, was depressed. Then one day she went to a lecture by an exercise physiologist who recommended people with problems such as hers to go running, starting with simple walking and progressing via fast walking to jogging. Despite never really having been one for exercise, she decided to go for it. Now, many years later, Mavis has run more than twenty marathons, her last one completed in a little over four hours – not bad for an eighty-two-year-old. She no longer has lung problems and is a model of fitness. Simply by changing the environment of her life she knocked twenty-five years off her biological age.

Genes and the Environment

Mavis's story is a good illustration of how the environment of your life – being the sum total of everything you eat, drink, breathe, think and exercise – can over-ride your genetic 'program'. This is both good news and bad news. The good news is that you, not your parents, are in charge of your own health. The bad news is that many hard-to-avoid factors in the modern environment can have an impact on how your genes express themselves and can affect your health and experience of life.

To illustrate how this works, consider the example of the chemical nonylphenol, found in paints, detergents, lubricating oils, toiletries, spermicide foams, agrochemicals and many other products. Inside our cells are receptors for hormones (see diagram overleaf). The hormone and receptor fit like lock and key. If the key fits, specific genes are activated, turning on a particular biological program. Fake hormones, such as nonylphenols, are like wonky keys. They can activates genes, but not necessarily the right ones, so they change the way our biology works. Nonylphenol is known as an oestrogen-mimicker and, like oestrogen itself, can change the programing of the body's biochemistry, depending on how much and what else your cells are exposed to.

The soya bean also contains an oestrogen-like molecule; however, in this case it seems to bind to oestrogen receptors and stop harmful substances like nonylphenols from perverting the course of genetics expression. So, if anything, it helps to balance hormones, while substances like nonylphenols disrupt normal hormone balance.

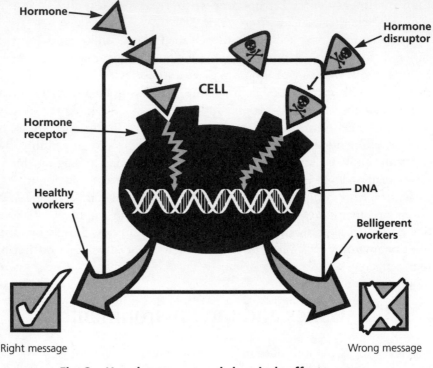

Fig. 3   How hormones and chemicals affect genes

Your total environmental load is determined by the balance between a long list of beneficial substances, mainly nutrients and natural food components, and a long and growing list of detrimental substances, mainly manmade. If you can deal with the load you stay healthy; if you're having difficulty you get sick; and if the load is just too much you die. The genetic strength you have inherited from your parents, plus your current biological function (the net result of your life's experiment so far) determine just how great a load you can bear before the camel's back breaks.

FOUR

REDEFINING HEALTH

Medicine as we know it defines health as 'an absence of illness'. You're tired all the time, you get headaches, you can't concentrate and you don't digest your food well – but the doctor says the tests are OK, you don't have high blood pressure, your cholesterol's fine, there's nothing to worry about. You're healthy.

But health is much more than this. Health is consistent energy, mental clarity, resistance to stress, freedom from infections, emotional balance, healthy skin, hair and nails, good physical strength and stamina, ageless ageing and . . . an absence of illness.

Most of what we know as healthcare is, in fact, disease care. The same applies to our 'health' service and 'health' insurance. They're not for healthy people, they're for diseased people. They cater for what you could call the horizontally ill – the bed-bound. Once they get the horizontally ill vertical again, the job's over. This is crisis medicine.

But what about all those who are neither ill nor 100 per cent healthy – the vertically ill: still walking, still going to work, but certainly not feeling great or functioning optimally, and probably experiencing some level of pain, tiredness and depression?

Functional Medicine

A new phrase has entered medical dictionaries in the 1990s – 'functional medicine'. It means the science of keeping people functioning at their full potential. It asks the question, 'What set of circumstances is needed for an individual to experience life fully?' Function is defined by the person. We know when we're functioning, when our mind is sharp or our body fit. One client defined health as being 'blissfully unaware of my body – free from pain'.

The concept of functional medicine, first coined by Dr Jeffrey Bland, grew out of twice Nobel Prize winner Dr Linus Pauling's vision of tomorrow's medicine. Having made numerous scientific contributions to modern medicine (not least of which was discovering how anaesthetics work, leading to the development of modern anaesthesia), he came to realise that the future of medicine lay in giving an individual the right nutrients to allow his or her body chemistry to function properly. He called this 'orthomolecular medicine' ('ortho' means 'right'), which became popularly known as 'optimum nutrition'. It poses the key question 'What do we need to eat, drink and breathe to realise our full potential?' Of course, for a truly holistic perspective one must add into the 'functional health' equation exercise and posture as well as mental, emotional and spiritual dimensions.

What Is Health?

From this perspective, health is a positive state of wellness, with all cylinders firing – not just a lack of illness. It's an ability to adapt positively to the changing circumstances of our lives.

Symptoms such as allergies, inflammation, pain, headaches, exhaustion, depression, tension, indigestion and recurrent infections are all signs that the individual isn't adapting to his environment. These symptoms, and conditions such as chronic fatigue syndrome, are classic responses to an overload of drugs, toxic chemicals, pollution, poor-quality food or allergy-provoking foods. With this understanding we can say that:

- **Health** is the ability to adapt to the environment and maintain optimal function.

- **Vertical Illness** is the ability to adapt partially to the environment, with a partial loss of function.

- **Horizontal Illness** is the inability to adapt to the environment, with a significant loss of function.

How healthy are you? Are you 100 per cent healthy, with consistent energy, a clear mind, and freedom from pain and infections? Or are you a long way short of your full potential? The Functional Health Questionnaire opposite can help show where you are on the scale of what's possible and help define the areas for improvement.

FUNCTIONAL HEALTH QUESTIONNAIRE

How healthy are you? Answer each of the following questions by circling **a**, **b** or **c** as appropriate, then see how you score at the end.

Digestion

Do you suffer from indigestion?
- **a** Frequently
- **b** Sometimes
- **c** Rarely or never

Do you suffer from bloatedness or flatulance?
- **a** Frequently
- **b** Sometimes
- **c** Rarely or never

Do you get sleepy after meals?
- **a** Frequently
- **b** Sometimes
- **c** Rarely or never

Do you get constipated?
- **a** Frequently
- **b** Sometimes
- **c** Rarely or never

Do you suffer from colitis, irritable bowel syndrome etc.?
- **a** Frequently
- **b** Sometimes
- **c** Rarely or never

Cardiovascular System

What is your blood pressure?
- **a** 140/90 or above
- **b** Between 125/85 and 140/90
- **c** Less than 125/85

If you don't know what your blood pressure is, get your doctor to check it and then include it in your score.

Do you get out of breath easily?
- **a** Frequently
- **b** Sometimes
- **c** Rarely or never

Do you get cold hands and feet?
   a Frequently
   b Sometimes
   c Rarely or never

Do you have a diagnosed circulatory problem?
   a Yes
   c No

How many of your parents, grandparents, uncles and aunts have died from cardio-vascular problems?
   a More than 3
   b 2
   c 1 or none

Immune System

How many colds do you get a year?
   a 3 or more
   b 2
   c 1 or none

How many days, on average, do the full symptoms of your colds last?
   a 3 or more
   b 2
   c 1 (or none if you get no colds)

How many times a year, on average, do you take a course of antibiotics?
   a 2 or more
   b 1
   c 0

Do you suffer from health problems that involve inflammation (pain and redness) (see p. 84)?
   a Yes
   c No

Do you often have allergic reactions?
   a Yes
   b Occasionally
   c No

Mental Health

Is your concentration poorer than it used to be?
   a Frequently
   b Sometimes
   c Rarely or never

Is your memory poorer than it used to be?
  a Frequently
  b Sometimes
  c Rarely or never

Do you get depressed?
  a Frequently
  b Sometimes
  c Rarely or never

Do you get anxious?
  a Frequently
  b Sometimes
  c Rarely or never

Do you have any diagnosed mental health problems?
  a Yes
  c No

Hormonal System

Do you suffer from PMS or menopausal symptoms?
  a Frequently
  b Sometimes
  c Rarely or never

Are your periods irregular or heavy and painful?
  a Frequently
  b Sometimes
  c Rarely or never

Do you get energy dips and crave sweet foods or stimulants?
  a Frequently
  b Sometimes
  c Rarely or never

Would you describe your lifestyle as stressful?
  a Frequently
  b Sometimes
  c Rarely or never

Do you need a stimulant or something sweet to get you going in the morning?
  a Frequently
  b Sometimes
  c Rarely or never

Skin, Nails and Hair

Do you have dry skin?
  a Frequently
  b Sometimes
  c Rarely or never

Do you get acne?
  a Frequently
  b Sometimes
  c Rarely or never

Do you get eczema, psoriasis or dermatitis?
  a Frequently
  b Sometimes
  c Rarely or never

Do you get weak, brittle or cracked nails?
  a Frequently
  b Sometimes
  c Rarely or never

Do you get dull, oily, or dry and brittle hair?
  a Frequently
  b Sometimes
  c Rarely or never

Physical Function

On average, how many times a week do you exercise?
  a Rarely or never
  b Once
  c Twice or more

How often do you strain a muscle when you exert yourself physically?
  a Frequently
  b Sometimes
  c Rarely or never

Do you sleep less than 6½ hours a night?
  a Frequently
  b Sometimes
  c Rarely or never

How often do you feel tired?
  a Frequently
  b Sometimes
  c Rarely or never

How often do you exercise?
   a Rarely or never
   b Sometimes
   c Frequently

Medical History

How many times a year do you visit your doctor?
   a 2 or more
   b Once
   c None

On average, how many drug prescriptions do you take each year?
   a 2 or more
   b 1
   c None

Are you . . . ?
   a Obese
   b Overweight
   c Ideal weight

How often were you ill as a child?
   a Frequently
   b Sometimes
   c Rarely or never

Do you have a current chronic health problem?
   a Yes
   c No

> Score 2 points for each **a** answer
>
> Score 1 point for each **b** answer
>
> Score 0 points for each **c** answer

The maximum score is 80. If you score . . .

80–51   You are 'vertically ill' and heading for horizontality unless you make some changes to your diet and lifestyle. See a nutrition consultant to find out what diet and supplement programme will restore your health reserve.

50–31   You are in average poor health and, unless you make some positive changes now, you can expect a gradually decreasing health reserve, resulting in problems later in life. See a nutrition consultant and fine-tune your diet.

30–15   You are in better than average health, but still below your potential. It's time to go one step further and improve your diet and lifestyle. Focus on the high-scoring questions and sections.

15–0   You're functionally healthy, with enough reserve to adapt to the stresses of life. High-scoring questions show you which areas need some attention.

Genes or Environment?

Assuming there's room for improvement, how are you going to achieve this? There are only two options: change your genes (the program you're born with) or change the environment of your life. Right now, the former is not possible. But you can change the way your genes express themselves. So that leaves one option, if you want to transform your health and, through that, your experience of life: change your environment. This does-n't mean moving house. It means taking an inventory of every outside fac-tor that affects your body and mind. This includes everything listed below:

Your chemical environment
- Intake of nutrients
- Intake of chemicals in food
- Intake of drugs
- Intake of alcohol
- Intake of cigarette smoke, including other people's
- Exposure to fumes and other air-borne pollutants
- Use of skin-penetrating chemicals in cosmetics, toiletries and household products
- Quantity and quality of water that you drink

Your physical environment
- Quantity and quality of exercise
- Quantity and quality of leisure
- Quantity and quality of sleep
- Level of physical tension

Your psychological environment
- Sources and level of stress
- Time pressures and management
- Opportunities for emotional expression
- Opportunities for creative expression
- Social and psychological support

Your Total Environmental Load

Most health problems are the consequence of an accumulation of stresses that eventually tip the body into overload. Long before there are noticeable symptoms, your body, struggling to adapt, starts to function differently, as if going on red alert. Then, as soon as the total environmental load is too great, your health breaks down. By the time you are in pain, have inflammation, headaches, exhaustion, allergies or frequent infections, you will have been living beyond your adaptive capacity in a state of red alert for some time. The final straw that triggers symptoms is not the cause of the disease, but just the last piece in a complex set of circumstances that lead to disease.

Consider the case of Anna, a young girl who is prone to asthma attacks when her parents argue. In the old way of thinking Anna will either be given a bronchodilating drug to suppress the symptoms, or her parents will be recommended counselling, or both. In the new way of thinking, her parents arguing is just the final straw, the trigger, which obviously needs to be addressed. But so too does the fact that she is deficient in vitamins, minerals and essential fatty acids, living in a polluted environment, showing signs of allergy to dairy produce, pollen and house dust mite, all of which predispose her to inflammatory reactions like asthma. Dealing with these factors makes her more able to adapt to her life circumstances without developing asthma.

Preventive Medicine

True preventive medicine is not about preventing disease by giving aspirin to thin the blood, or hormones to stop osteoporosis. It's about keeping people close to 100 per cent health, in which disease is not a possibility, in which the body has plenty of reserve, operating well within its adaptive capacity. That's the purpose of the rest of this book: to give you concrete ways to make adjustments to your diet, lifestyle and way of thinking to close the gap between how you are now and your true potential. Even minor changes to your diet, lifestyle or the way you influence your children can have profound effects. For example:

- Breastfeeding a baby dramatically reduces the risk of ear infections in the first three years, and cancer later in life,[10] as well as reducing the risk of developing allergies.[11]

- Deep breathing exercises halve the incidence of hot flushes in menopausal women.[12]

- A mile run or walked adds twenty-one minutes to your life and saves 20p in medical care.[13]

- Thirty minutes of T'ai Chi markedly improves your immune strength.[14]

- A daily multivitamin halves the incidence of infections among the elderly.[15]

- One gram of vitamin C significantly lowers high blood pressure[16] and reduces the incidence, duration and severity of colds.[17]

- A carrot a day halves your risk of a stroke and reduces cholesterol.[18]

- Broccoli, Brussels sprouts or cabbage[19] or garlic and onions[20] every day halves your risk of stomach cancer, while a tomato a day cuts a man's risk of prostate cancer by 20 per cent.[21]

- Eating foods rich in antioxidants has a greater effect in reducing cancer risk than not smoking.[22]

These are a tiny fraction of the number of positive health tips gleaned from recent medical research. This book will help you to identify which ones can take you towards 100 per cent health. Aren't a few simple changes to your diet and lifestyle a small price to pay for adding years to your life and life to your years?

FIVE

ADAPTING TO THE
TWENTY-FIRST CENTURY

There's an old Chinese curse which runs: 'May you live in interesting times.' As we turn the corner into the twenty-first century these are certainly interesting times, with rapid change including the globalisation of markets, information and ideas. Old cultures and traditions that may have stayed the same for centuries are having to adapt radically or die out. Complexity and change challenge us every day.

Interestingly, the nature of the diseases we now face seem to reflect the times we live in. Less significant now are the diseases of the eighteenth and nineteenth century such as tuberculosis, scarlet fever, rheumatic fever, diptheria and cholera which accounted for the majority of deaths in an era when freedom of expression was curtailed, when women were bound by a strictly male-dominated society with strict codes of behaviour, and when that society had a rigid class structure.

Instead, our diseases are now those of body systems gone haywire, of an inability to adapt: cancer, allergies, chronic fatigue syndrome, osteoporosis, endometriosis, diabetes, asthma, irritable bowel syndrome, obesity, depression and anxiety. It's as if many modern diseases reflect the loss of control experienced in these rapidly changing times.

The Neuro-Endo-Immune Network

Like the times we live in, modern diseases are proving to be complex, with interactions between different systems of the body. Increasing evidence is linking three adaptive systems of the body – the nervous system (including the brain), the immune system and the endocrine system (which produces hormones). All three systems may indeed be one neuro-endo-immune network that helps us to adapt to our world.

Each of these systems 'talk'. The brain and nervous system talk via

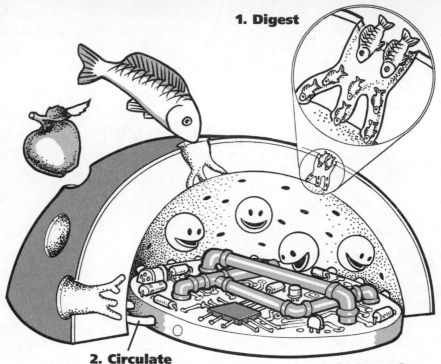

1. Digest

2. Circulate

3. Organise

The neuro-endo-immune network interlinks the brain and nervous system *(electronic circuit)*, the immune system *(pacmen)* and the hormone-producing endocrine system *(plumbing)*.
Across this network everything you see, touch, taste, or smell is processed – giving rise to the emotional, physical and chemical responses you call your life.

Fig. 4

neurotransmitters, special chemicals that cross between neuron cells, triggering the passing of an electrical message. These neurotransmitters are made from amino acids and their function is controlled by phospholipids, special fats that help insulate and control the electrical messages.

The endocrine system talks with hormones. These are produced in special cells and enter the bloodstream, by which they travel to cells and give them instructions. Hormones are made from amino acids or special fat compounds called steroids.

The immune system talks via immune cells, whose main component is protein. Some of these cells are antibodies, made out of amino acids and capable of responding to undesirable substances.

Each system is fundamentally affected by what you eat. Amino acids, essential fats, vitamins and minerals are all needed to produce neurotransmitters, hormones and immune cells. With this in mind, human anatomy and physiology can be reorganised into three fundamental processes:

Digestion

Receiving and digesting the right nutrients is the first prerequisite for health. Since we are made from what we eat, not eating the right foods or not digesting them well means that no system of the body can receive the right supplies to carry out its job properly.

Circulation

The transport of these nutrients is the next step: that means getting nutrients to the cells and taking away the garbage. Blockages in the arteries or poor delivery of oxygen (perhaps due to insufficient protective antioxidants or a lack of iron or vitamin B12) are just two examples of a poor delivery service. Eating the wrong foods (excess protein, perhaps) results in too many toxic by-products. These can heavily tax the body's recycling plant, the liver, and lead to the 'dumping' of toxins in fat cells.

Organisation

This is the single most complex function within the body. Only living systems can continually remake and reorganise themselves, to maintain order and adapt to an ever-changing environment. This process is called homeodynamics. Very little in you was there last year, yet your body gives the semblance of continuity and integrity. This 'adapting' process is masterminded by the neuro-endo-immune network, described as a network because there is evidence of complex communication facilitating continual adaptation, rather like the organisation of a society or a community. This network is intelligent, working for the whole. It is a complex adaptive system.

Your health hinges on taking in the right molecules, digesting and absorbing them, then circulating them to supply the neuro-endo-immune network with amino acids, fats, vitamins and minerals – in other words, fuel, building materials and communication tools. You are the guardian of this highly intelligent system – your body.

PART 2

THE MEDICINE OF TOMORROW

Healthcare today is the fastest-growing failing business.

DR EMANUEL CHERASKIN

SIX

NUTRACEUTICALS VS PHARMACEUTICALS

The financial foundation of the pharmaceutical industry lies in developing man-made chemicals which can be patented. The patent guarantees the company exclusive rights to market the drug usually for a period of fifteen years at the price they choose. On this basis, investment is made to test, prove and market a drug for a particular use, all of which normally costs around £100 million.

Naturally occurring substances cannot be patented. For this reason it is much less profitable to exploit the medicinal power of something like vitamin C. Anyone can sell it, and market forces work to keep the price down.

AZT is one of the most popular drugs for the treatment of HIV infection. The cost of the recommended daily dose (500mg) is £6.25 or $10. That's £190 a month. Vitamin C has proved more effective than AZT in suppressing HIV in infected human cells. The cost of 20,000mg a day, the highest recommended dose, is 58p or 90c. That's £18 a month. So, in this case, the pharmaceutical AZT is ten times more expensive than vitamin C. This dramatic difference in cost is not uncommon. Drugs are expensive and that's why the UK National Health Service drug bill is £4.3 billion per annum, roughly £71 per person.

The other problem with pharmaceuticals like AZT is that most have side-effects because they are not natural and have not been part of the evolution of the body's chemical systems. Vitamin C, however, has formed part of this evolution; it has no known toxicity unless injected in massive amounts. Most substances, including water, are toxic if taken in large enough amounts. Nutraceuticals (nutrients like vitamin C that are part of our evolutionary design) tend to be much better tolerated than man-made drugs.

When effectiveness, toxicity and cost are taken into account, many nutraceuticals outperform common pharmaceuticals, especially when they form part of an overall dietary programme. Some of the most promising nutraceuticals are shown below and are well worth trying if you suffer from any of these health problems.

Disease or Symptom	Common Drugs	Best Nutraceuticals
Anxiety	Benzodiazepine tranquillisers (Diazepam, Temazepam)	• B complex, folic acid • Calcium, magnesium and zinc
Arthritis	NSAIDs, or Non-Steroidal Anti-Inflammatory Drugs (Ibuprofen, Diclofenac), Cortisone (Prednisolone)	• Evening primrose oil and fish oils • Boswellic acid • Glucosamine
Asthma	Bronchodilators (Salbutamol, Ventolin)	• Evening primrose oil and fish oils • Vitamins A, C and antioxidants (eliminate allergies)
Colds & flu	Decongestants (Sudafed)	• Vitamin C, zinc and antioxidants • Elderberry extract, Cat's Claw, Echinacea
Depression	Antidepressants (Prozac, Amitriptyline)	• Vitamins B3, B12 and folic acid • Tryptophan, Tyrosine
Eczema	Corticosteroid creams	• Evening primrose oil and fish oils • Vitamin C, magnesium, zinc (eliminate allergies)
Headache	Painkillers (Aspirin, Paracetamol)	• Vitamin B3 as niacin • Digestive enzymes
Heart disease	Aspirin, Calcium blocker (Istin)	• Vitamins C and E plus B3 • EPA/DHA from fish oils • Lysine
High blood pressure	Aspirin, Beta-blockers (Atenolol), Antihypertensive (Enalapril)	• Vitamins C and E plus B3 • EPA/DHA from fish oils
Infections	Antibiotics (Penicillin, Amoxycillin)	• Vitamin C, zinc and antioxidants • Elderberry extract, Cat's Claw, Echinacea
Insomnia	Sleeping pills (Mogadon, Xanax)	• Vitamins B3, B6 and C • Calcium, magnesium and zinc • Tryptophan
PMS and Menopausal Problems	HRT (Premarin)	• Vitamins E, B6, zinc and magnesium • Evening primrose oil • Natural progesterone

Food as Medicine

By far the most important source of nutraceuticals is food, not supplements. Many natural foods provide over twenty active nutraceuticals in significant enough quantities to make a real difference to your health.

Consider the cruciferous family of vegetables – cabbage, broccoli, Brussels sprouts and cauliflower. Apart from the many vitamins and minerals they contain they provide large amounts of glucosinolates which are proving to be very powerful health-promoting nutrients. Not only does the consumption of these foods reduce your risk of cancer substantially – three servings a week cuts your risk of getting colon cancer by 60 per cent, for example – but they also increase the body's ability to deal with toxins. Glucosinolates have been shown to improve liver detoxification potential by 30 per cent if you eat the equivalent of three servings of these vegetables a day. So here is a common food which not only reduces your risk of disease but also improves your adaptive capacity. Many other foods, such as carrots, tomatoes, soya beans and garlic, are showing equivalent effects.

Instead of using pharmaceutical drugs with undesirable side-effects the medicine of tomorrow is turning to nutraceuticals, nature's pharmacy of nutrients, supplied as food and supplements, to correct the body's chemistry and restore wellbeing.

SEVEN

PROBIOTICS vs ANTIBIOTICS

Up to 2kg of your body weight consists of bacteria. The average person is host to around four hundred different types of friendly bacteria, mainly resident in the digestive tract, which are forever multiplying. These 'good' bacteria are the first line of defence against unfriendly (pathogenic) bacteria and other disease-producing microbes, including viruses and fungi. They also make some vitamins and digest fibre, allowing us to derive more nutrients from otherwise indigestible food.

We are, in fact, part-descended from bacteria. The energy factories within our cells, called mitochondria, are derived from bacteria. Biologists now believe that the complex cells that make up our body may have developed by 'working together' with smaller micro-organisms like bacteria. In time, this cooperation led to the development of the complex cells from which we are made.

Like pesticides, the purpose of antibiotic drugs is to kill life (anti-bio). But as well as destroying pathogenic bacteria, antibiotics also destroy friendly ones. The more 'broad-spectrum' the antibiotic, the more strains of beneficial bacteria will also be killed. A single course of antibiotics can wipe out beneficial strains of bacteria for six months or more. 'When you take antibiotics, you are doing to your body what a farmer does when he sprays his fields with pesticides,' says medical researcher Geoffrey Cannon, author of Superbug.[23]

Do Antibiotics Do More Harm Than Good?

According to microbiologist Professor Richard Lacey, the widespread overuse of antibiotics is the major cause of changes observed in the last decade in the balance of bacteria in the gut. Overuse of antibiotics, in particular ampicillin and tetracyclines, is resulting in a generation of new strains of 'superbugs' – bacteria which have become resistant to the very drugs designed to destroy them. Medical researcher Dr Stuart Levy from Tufts University in Boston says that these changes are 'unparalleled in recorded biologic history'. So serious is the problem that now there are new drug-resistant versions of every disease-causing bacterium. Drug-resistant tuberculosis, for example, now accounts for one in 7 new cases.

Antibiotics also have acute, short-term ill effects, ranging from rashes to diarrhoea, and long-term ill effects. The long-term effects are more worrying. Anyone taking broad-spectrum antibiotics continually over a period of years becomes extremely vulnerable to invasion by other bacterial species, fungi and viruses. According to Geoffrey Cannon 'antibiotics are implicated as a cause of new diseases that are in some way identified with bacteria not normally present in the body. Bacteria that have evolved with us are our outer immune defences, so it follows that anything you do that damages what is a very complex mircrobial ecology in the body must lay you open to other diseases.' He believes it is unwise to use antibiotics except in cases where there is real reason to believe that a bacterial infection is life-threatening or could lead to more serious illness if left unchecked.

Infection Epidemic Predicted

It is not just antibiotics, but the whole mentality of developing drugs to kill bugs that needs to be questioned. After all, vast improvements in sanitation in the Western world have been achieved this century, and in the last twenty years medicine has doled out billions of antibiotic, antiviral and antifungal medicines. If this approach was working you would expect fewer deaths overall from infections and fewer cases of food poisoning. In fact, exactly the opposite has occurred.

In both the USA and the UK the number of infections is dramatically on the increase. A survey of all deaths in the USA between 1980 and 1992 revealed an alarming 58 per cent increase in deaths from infectious diseases.[24] A sixfold increase occurred in those between the ages of twenty-five and forty-four. This is only partly due to the increased number of deaths from HIV infection. Deaths from respiratory infections increased by 20 per cent. The same trends are occurring in Britain, according to Spence Galbraith, former director of the Communicable Diseases Surveillance Centre,[25] 'The rate of change of human infection appears to be increasing. It is now recognised that it can only be a matter of time until the next microbial menace to our species emerges amongst us.'

Food Bugs – a Growing Problem

What of food poisoning? Has this been abetted by adding antibiotics to animal feed, by modern methods of farming, food processing and storing?

More than a million people are dying from food poisoning each year round the world.[26] Indeed, the growing incidence of disease caused by food bugs, now second only to the common cold in some Western countries, may already be one knock-on effect of the global use of around 50,000 tons of antibiotics each year.

The problem, in part, goes back to the post-war years when the demand for meat, a favourite home for pathogens, increased sharply. As a result the demand also increased for cheap animal feed from tropical countries, where animal infection is widespread. Although national legislation and inter-national codes have addressed this problem, the legacy remains. Animals given these contaminated feeds in turn contaminated the environment by enabling micro-organisms to establish themselves widely. Millions of animals from all over the world have contributed to this environmental problem and to the creation of infection cycles, which to this day play an important role in food-borne disease.

The problem is compounded by the structure of the modern food processing industry. For example, because processing plants are centralised a single infected animal could infect a whole city's meat supply. The decline in home cooking and the increase of mass catering through restaurants, fast-food outlets and ready-meals adds to the problem. This, combined with the growing number of people with weakened immune systems (partly due to the widespread use of drugs such as antibiotics) and the development of more drug-resistant strains of bacteria, is making the situation critical. High-risk foods are meat, eggs and dairy produce.

Know Your Enemy

The best way to fight infection is to have a strong immune system and the right balance of beneficial bacteria in the gut. Then if a pathogen does come along, your natural defences can probably fight it off. But what if you do succumb to an infection?

Contrary to popular belief, most illnesses are not infections and most infections are not best treated by antibiotics. Viral diseases, such as colds or flu, don't respond to antibiotics. Antibiotics don't work for sore throats either, according to a study published in the *British Medical Journal*.[27] Over seven hundred patients with sore throats were divided into three groups: some were given antibiotics for ten days, some were given antibiotics after three days if their symptoms had not cleared, and some were given nothing. There was no difference between the groups in the number of people feeling better after three days, nor in the overall length of illness.

Many simple gut infections like gastroenteritis or diarrhoea can actually get worse if treated with antibiotics, because beneficial and protective bacteria get destroyed too. Antibiotics should also never be used to prevent an infection, for example in the treatment of acne, as they weaken a person's immunity and leave them open to other infections. Professor Richard Lacey's recommendation is that doctors should test whether a sick person has a bacterial infection, identify the type of bacteria, prescribe an antibiotic specifically designed for it for as short a time as possible, and tell the patient to discontinue the course as soon as the symptoms go away.

Recent advances in analytical testing have made it possible to take a saliva or stool sample and identify any lurking pathogens. It is also possible to discover whether you're lacking any key beneficial bacteria, the body's natural defences.

Fighting Infections Naturally

These advances are leading practitioners towards the therapeutic use of probiotics (beneficial bacteria) and away from antibiotics. Instead of prescribing a drug to wipe out the enemy, specific strains of beneficial bacteria are given to reinforce the body's natural defences. For example, giving children probiotics had been shown to halve the recovery time from a bout of diarrhoea.

The principal friendly bacteria include the families of *Lactobacillus* and *Bifidus* bacteria. Supplementing these gives pathogenic bacteria less chance of survival. There are many different strains of friendly bacteria, some of which actually live in the gut, while others simply pass through and are useful while they're there. Here are some of the different types:

The Principal Friendly Bacteria

	Children	Adults
Resident	B. infantis	L. acidophilus
	B. bifidum	B. bacterium
		L. salivarius
		Enterococci
Passing through	L. bulgaricus	L. casei (from cheese)
	S. thermophilus	S. thermophilus
		L. salivarius
		L. bulgaricus

Key
B. = Bifidobacteria   L. = Lactobacillus   S. = Streptococcus

Those that are resident, sometimes called 'human strain', are usually more powerful at fighting infection. Others are available in fermented foods such as yoghurt, miso and sauerkraut. Health food stores stock probiotic supplements, many of which contain a combination of beneficial bacteria. Ask for advice on the best one to take, depending on your circumstances. Generally, you need to take one or two capsules, or a teaspoon, every day, providing in the order of a billion individual bacteria. It's best to take them with food if the bacteria are micro-encapsulated; otherwise take them away from meals to minimise their destruction from gastric acid in the stomach.

Nature's pharmacy is also rich in natural infection fighters, from grapefruit seed extract to the herb artemisia. Both of these can also help to get rid of harmful microbes without upsetting healthy intestinal flora.

The chart below shows which natural medicines and strains of beneficial bacteria are most effective against specific kinds of infections. Used in combination, these can be very powerful. You may need to seek the advice of a nutrition consultant (see p. 210) for a specific strategy against more serious infections. As a general rule, if an infection has persisted for more than a week and has not responded to these combinations you should see your doctor. In some cases antibiotics are necessary, but they should only be used as a last resort. If they are, be sure to take a course of probiotics such as *Lactobacillus acidophilus* and *bifidus* for one month to restore your healthy gut bacteria.

Fighting Infections Naturally

Infection	Natural Medicine/Beneficial Bacteria
Stomach bugs and traveller's diarrhoea (holidays)	grapefruit seed (ST), garlic, iodine (ST), Lactobacillus acidophilus, bifidobacteria, aloe vera
Diarrhoea	grapefruit seed (ST), L. infantis (kids), avoid milk due to bacteria, induced lactase deficiency, lactose free
Food poisoning	Lactobacillus acidophilus, garlic, aloe vera
Sore throats, tonsillitis, laryngitis	vitamin C plus bioflavonoids, vitamin A, zinc, acidophilus, bee propolis, garlic, elderberry extract (Sambucol), cat's claw (NP&ST)
Bronchitis	vitamin C with bioflavonoids, zinc, vitamin A, echinacea (NP&ST), elderberry extract (Sambucol), essential fatty acids
Sinusitis	vitamin C, zinc, eucalyptus inhalation, bee pollen, zinc, cat's claw (NP&ST)

Colds & flu	vitamin C with bioflavonoids, vitamin A, elderberry extract (Sambucol), cat's claw (NP&ST)
Ear infections	vitamins A, C and E, zinc, manganese, garlic, grapefruit seed drops (ST)
Eye infections	vitamins A and C, zinc, bilberry, essential fats
Candidiasis	caprylic acid (NP), oleic acid, artemisia, garlic, grapefruit seed extract (ST), black barberry (burberine) (ST, NP)
Anti-parasites	artemisia, grapefruit seed extract (ST)
Athlete's foot	garlic, vitamin C, acidophilus, essential fats
Herpes Simplex	L-lysine, vitamins A and C, zinc, L. bulgaricus

Remember, just because something's natural doesn't mean it's harmless. Those remedies marked 'ST' are for short-term use only, either because they're only useful for fighting a current infection or because long-term use (more than a month) may not be advantageous. Some herbs contain alkaloids or other substances that could, in high dose, be harmful in pregnancy. Those marked 'NP' are best not taken if you are pregnant.

Strengthen Your Defences

There's plenty you can do to keep your defences strong so as to avoid getting an infection in the first place. The first thing is to make sure you're eating good food. The key immune-boosting nutrients are vitamins A, C and B6, and minerals such as magnesium and zinc. The vast majority of people fail to get even Recommended Daily Allowance (RDA) levels of these nutrients from their diet, let alone optimal intakes. For this reason supplementing a good, all-round, high-strength multivitamin is a proven way to boost your defences. In a double-blind, controlled trial, elderly people who took a multivitamin halved their number of infections and had measurable improvements in the strength of their immune systems.[15]

Vitamin C is strongly antiviral and has proved successful against every virus tested so far, from HIV to the common cold.[28] The mineral zinc, in doses of 100mg a day, has also proved to be antiviral and is available in lozenges for coughs and colds.[29] This level is for short-term use only.

Here are a few tips to keep your immune system in top form:

● Eat five servings of fruit and vegetables every day. They contain many immune-boosting antioxidants and phytonutrients (beneficial chemicals found in plants).

- Eat less meat, eggs and dairy produce and be choosy about their source. Eat organic or free-range to avoid antibiotic residues, and check for freshness. Many eggs are four weeks old before you eat them. Avoid dairy products completely if you've got excessive mucus, e.g. sinus infection or cold.

- Alcohol, smoking, drugs, coffee, late nights, eating too much, working too hard and not getting enough sleep all deplete the immune system. Keep your overload down.

- Supplement 1000–2000mg of vitamin C every day, as well as a good all-round multivitamin and mineral containing at least 3300mcg vitamin A, 10mg B6, 15mg zinc and 100mcg selenium.

- At the first sign of a viral infection (e.g. cold or flu) increase your vitamin C intake to 3000mg every four hours; suck zinc lozenges; drink two cups of cat's claw tea a day (made from the loose herb brewed in water, not teabags, and add blackcurrant/apple juice concentrate for taste); and take four dessertspoons of black elderberry extract (Sambucol) a day.

- If on holiday in a place where you know hygiene standards are likely to be low, such as the Far East, take a probiotic supplement such as *Lactobacillus acidophilus* and *bifidus* daily to build up your beneficial bacteria. Also, carry grapefruit seed extract with you and take ten drops two or three times a day if you suspect an infection.

- Keep fit. Exercise, especially yoga and T'ai Chi, improve immunity. Don't over-exercise, though – too much weakens the immune system.

EIGHT

Neuroanalysis vs Psychoanalysis

According to the World Health Organisation, mental illness will be the most common major health issue in the twenty-first century. In the UK there are 6 million sufferers – that's roughly one in 10 people – and the numbers are rising. Mental problem debates usually revolve around whether the problem is psychological, in which case counselling is recommended, or chemical, in which case drugs are recommended.

Of course, life isn't black and white: mental health problems are often a combination of social and psychological factors, plus biochemical imbalances, which are sometimes partly genetic. These factors interweave, as illustrated by the story of David, who had suffered very real physical symptoms of chronic fatigue for five years. His doctor diagnosed him as being depressed and his symptoms as due to the depression, to which he replied, 'Of course I'm depressed. Wouldn't you be if you'd been exhausted for five years and unable to support yourself?' In his case neither drugs nor psychotherapy helped. What worked was a radical change in his diet, backed up by large quantities of specific vitamins and minerals to correct his particular biochemical imbalance.

Mind or Body?

There are several physical conditions which have repercussions on mental health. These include blood sugar problems, thyroid problems, adrenal exhaustion, chronic fatigue syndrome and viral infections. Tranquillisers and antidepressants certainly shouldn't be prescribed until these have been ruled out.

Then, of course, there are mental health problems resulting primarily from psychological problems. These respond best to psychotherapy or counselling, which has provided good results especially in cases of depression and anxiety.

Psychotherapy is not, however, so successful for those with problems such as abnormal perceptions and thought processes. Examples of these perceptual problems include seeing or hearing things, loss of body sensation, strange tastes or smells, disperceptions about body image, disturbed appetite, disturbed thinking processes, blank mind and the inability to concentrate. Such symptoms are often lumped together as schizophrenia, although some perceptual problems do occur in those diagnosed with attention deficit disorder, anorexia and manic depression.

A significant proportion of mentally unwell people fit into this category, and many respond neither to drugs nor to psychotherapy. This is perhaps because the primary cause of their problem is not a lack of drugs, nor a lack of psychological insight or support, but a chemical imbalance that affects how they think and feel. This can be brought on by years of inadequate nutrition and exposure to pollutants, drugs or environmental toxins.

To some people this idea may seem strange, almost too simplistic. Yet any intelligent person will recognise that our diets have changed fundamentally in the last hundred years, as too have the air we breathe, the water we drink and the environment in which we live. When we consider that the body and brain are made entirely from food, air and water, and that simple molecules like alcohol can fundamentally affect the brain, it is completely feasible that changes in diet and the environment have affected mental health.

Nutrition – the Forgotten Mental Health Factor

It is a surprising fact that nutritional intervention, involving improved diet plus large amounts of specific nutrients, has proved highly effective in treating acute schizophrenia,[30] attention deficit disorder,[31] anorexia,[32] delinquent and criminal behaviour,[33] depression[34,35] and insomnia.[36]

In double-blind controlled studies, Canadian psychiatrist Dr Abram Hoffer reported an 80 per cent remission from acute schizophrenia using vitamin B3 (niacin); Dr Birmingham of St Paul's Hospital, Vancouver, reported double the weight gain in anorexic patients given 50mg of zinc versus a placebo; Professor Stephen Schoenthaler at the University of California has shown that violations in prison communities can be halved by nutritional intervention: Dr Edward Reynolds at King's College Hospital in London has demonstrated improved recovery in depressed and schizophrenic patients with folic acid; and Dr Phillip Cowen from the University of Oxford's Department of Psychiatry has reported recovery from depression in people given the amino acid tryptophan, which is also well known for its effectiveness in treating insomnia.

Despite forty years of good clinical research, most psychiatrists continue to ignore these proven, safe approaches. Why? I am convinced that part of the reason is the way we conceive of 'mind' and 'body' as somehow separate. We tend to think of 'mind' as anything psychological – our thoughts and feelings – and of body as anything physical, including the brain. So, often a psychiatrist says, 'Is it psychological, in which case I'll recommend counselling – or is it a brain chemistry problem, in which case I'll recommend a drug.' Yet if you were to ask a biochemist and a psychologist to define where the mind starts and the body ends, they would find that the two were closely interconnected.

The intricate functioning of the neuro-endo-immune network (see Chapter 5) affects our overall health, not least our mental state. The slightest imbalance in the systems – nervous, immune and endocrine – can manifest itself mentally in anything from a little grumpiness to severe depression. It follows, therefore, that our mental state is fundamentally bound to these three body systems, whose optimal function depends, in turn, on nutritional factors. We all know how having a bit too much to drink can affect someone's mood the next day, but that's just an obvious example. The general balance of the neuro-endo-immune network is much more subtle than that: it relies on an intricate set of cofactors – vitamins, minerals, amino acids and fats – which we can get from our food.

Redefining Mind

In the context of this model the 'mind' is clearly not the brain. Intelligent 'conversations' are taking place at every moment across this network that runs throughout our body. This would explain why you can have a 'gut feeling' or 'heartache' or why your immune system becomes depressed when you are grieving. Mental processes, be they conscious like a thought, or unconscious like an instinctive fear reaction, are like ripples across the network, changing our balance of hormones, nervous system activity and immunity.

So 'mind' doesn't exist anywhere – it is the pattern of activity that occurs across this network. It is more like the program, the software-in-action. The hardware is the body, including the components of the neuro-endo-immune network such as nerve cells, neurotransmitters, immune cells, antibodies and hormones. These are made from food, so without the right food components there's no way mental processes will work properly. This would explain why, for example, counselling of young offenders becomes much more effective once their nutrition is improved.[37]

Neuroanalysis

With this view in mind, the first tenet of modern psychiatry should be to check that a person's neuro-endo-immune network is functioning properly. This can be done from the outside in or the inside out. From the outside in means checking that the person is receiving the right intake of nutrients, be they essential fats, vitamins, minerals or amino acids, and not taking in anti-nutrients such as drugs, pollutants, toxins, stimulants and excess sugar. From the inside out means checking whether the person actually has a hormonal, immune or neurotransmitter imbalance.

The whole of modern, drug-oriented psychiatry is based on the concept that some people have such neurotransmitter imbalances. An excess of dopamine or adrenalin is linked to mania and schizophrenia. Deficiency of these and of serotonin, another neurotransmitter, is linked to depression. The principle of antidepressants and tranquillisers is to interfere with these vital brain chemicals. For example the most popular 'serotonin-reuptake inhibitor', Prozac, aims to treat depression by increasing serotonin levels; it does this by preventing its natural breakdown in the body.

Yet before drugs are prescribed few if any patients are ever tested for evidence of a deficiency or excess of these neurotransmitters. Such neuro-analysis would identify much more precisely whether it really is an underlying biochemical imbalance that is tipping a person over into depression or anxiety states.

Nutrients Work Better Than Drugs

Of course, drugs aren't the only way to 'tune' your neurotransmitters. Take serotonin, for example, a lack of which is related to insomnia and depression. Instead of taking a drug to stop the body breaking down serotonin, why not change your diet to encourage the body to make more? This is the question that Dr Phillip Cowen from Oxford University set out to investigate.[38] Since serotonin is made from the amino acid tryptophan he placed fifteen women who had recovered from depression on a diet low in tryptophan. Within hours five had a full recurrence of their depression, five had a partial recurrence, and overall there was a significant increase in their depression rating. Conversely, giving tryptophan has been shown to relieve depression.[39]

For the body to turn tryptophan into serotonin, vitamins B3, B6 and zinc are essential. The combination of these nutrients may prove to be a highly effective way of helping people who are prone to depression or insomnia due to serotonin deficiency. Other amino acids, in combination with vitamins and minerals, are also proving helpful for a wide variety of mental health problems.

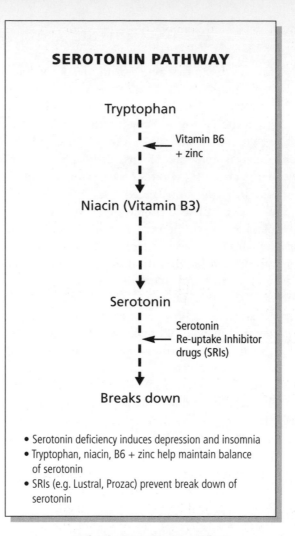

SEROTONIN PATHWAY

Tryptophan

Vitamin B6 + zinc

Niacin (Vitamin B3)

Serotonin

Serotonin Re-uptake Inhibitor drugs (SRIs)

Breaks down

- Serotonin deficiency induces depression and insomnia
- Tryptophan, niacin, B6 + zinc help maintain balance of serotonin
- SRIs (e.g. Lustral, Prozac) prevent break down of serotonin

Which Nutrients Help?

Depression   vitamin B complex, especially B3, B12 and folic acid; magnesium and tryptophan

Insomnia   vitamins B6, B3 and C, calcium, magnesium, zinc and chromium

Anxiety   vitamin B complex, especially folic acid; vitamin C, calcium and magnesium

Schizophrenia   vitamin B complex, especially B3, B12 and folic acid; vitamin C, zinc, calcium, magnesium and methionine

Anorexia   vitamin B complex, zinc, magnesium, amino acid complex

Attention Deficit Disorder vitamins B3, B6 and C, magnesium, calcium, zinc and essential fats

The other advantage of rebalancing the neuro-endo-immune network with nutrients rather than with drugs is that the former have fewer side-effects. Antidepressants and tranquillisers are alien substances to the brain and body and often introduce a wobble into the neuro-endo-immune network, experienced as side-effects. Nutrients are not alien and consequently much safer. Renowned mental health expert Dr Carl Pfeiffer, who spent fifty years researching the biochemistry of mental illness, said, 'If there's a drug that can alter brain chemistry for good effect, there's a nutrient that can do it without side-effects.' He, like other psychiatrists who have experimented with nutritional approaches to mental illness, rarely resorted to drugs, achieving better results with specific nutrient programmes.

So here are some general guidelines to keep yourself in good mental health:

- Avoid sugar and refined goods

- Eat more fresh fruit, vegetables and whole foods (e.g. seeds, nuts, beans, lentils and wholegrains)

- Avoid or reduce stimulants (i.e. tea, coffee, chocolate, cola drinks and cigarettes)

- Avoid or reduce alcohol. The consumption of alcohol increases your potential for allergies

- Have a heaped teaspoon of ground seeds (sesame, sunflower, pumpkin or flax), or a tablespoon of their oil, every day.

Most habits take a month to break. So take one habit, like drinking coffee. Give yourself one month without it, then see how you feel. The healthier your diet, the less extreme will be the withdrawal effects of these stimulants. The greater the withdrawal effects you experience, the worse this substance is for you. Take one step at a time and know that every step makes a difference.

Supplements for Mental Health

The brain uses about a third of all the nutrients we take in from our food. The following recommendations are for anyone who wants to promote and maintain their mental health:

- Supplement your diet with a high-strength multivitamin supplement containing vitamins A, B, C, D and E. Make sure your supplement contains at least 75mg niacin, pantothenic acid (B5) and pyridoxine, at least 100mcg folic acid (unless you are histadelic and experiencing mental health problems), and 10mcg B12.

- Supplement between 1000mg and 3000mg of vitamin C every day.

- Supplement a high-strength multimineral providing at least 400mg calcium, 200mg magnesium, 15mg zinc, 5mg manganese, 100mcg chromium and 100mcg selenium.

- Unless you are eating seeds and/or their oils most days, consider supplementing omega-6 oils such as evening primrose or borage (sometimes known as starflower) oil and omega-3 oils from flax seed (also known as linseed) or fish oils.

If you are suffering from a mental health problem it is best to see a nutrition consultant or nutritionally oriented psychiatrist, who can assess your nutrient status and neurotransmitter levels before recommending a nutritionally based strategy appropriate to your needs.

PART 3

WOMEN'S HEALTH REVOLUTION

The widespread prescribing of synthetic hormones to women was the biggest medical bungle this century.

KATE NEIL

HORMONES IN HAVOC

Something is seriously amiss with our hormones. Over the last fifty years there's been an undeniable escalation of hormone-related health problems. The incidence of infertility, fibroids, endometriosis, polycystic breasts, and ovarian, cervical and breast cancer has increased steadily and dramatically. Breast cancer incidence, for example, has almost tripled, affecting one in 8 women in Britain at some time in their life, compared to one in 22 in the 1940s.[40,41]

And the problem doesn't just relate to women. Male sperm count has dropped by 50 per cent in fifty years.[42] Rates of testicular and prostate cancer, as well as benign prostatic enlargement are up.[43,44] The incidence of males born with genital defects and of boys with undescended testes has doubled.[45,46]

In one of the most extraordinary detective stories of our times (documented in two excellent books, *Our Stolen Future* and *The Feminisation of Nature*, details of which are given on p. 202), leading scientists from many disciplines have come to the same conclusions. 'We've released chemicals throughout the world that are having fundamental effects on the reproductive system and immune system in wildlife and humans,' says Professor Louis Guillette of the University of Florida. 'We have unwittingly entered the ultimate Faustian bargain ... In return for all the benefits of our modern society, and all the amazing products of modern life, we have more testicular cancer and more breast cancer. We may also affect the ability of the species to reproduce,' says Devra Lee Davis, former deputy health policy adviser to the US government.

They and countless other scientists believe that a growing number of commonly occurring chemicals found in air, water and food are disrupting hormone balances and altering the course of nature. These hormone-disrupting chemicals include:

- **Pesticides:** DDT, DDE, endosulfan, methoxychlor, heptachlor, toxaphene, dieldrin, Lindane

- **Plastic compounds:** alkyphenols, such as nonylphenol and octylphenol; bisphenolic compounds, such as bisphenol A; phthalates

- **Industrial compounds:** some PCBs, dioxin, plus those listed for plastics

- **Pharmaceutical drugs:** synthetic oestrogens, such as DES

Most of these substances mimic the role played in the body by oestrogen, a hormone that stimulates the growth of hormone-sensitive tissue. When absorbed on top of the natural oestrogen produced by both men and women, plus the added oestrogen taken in by women on the pill or HRT, these chemicals can 'over-oestrogenise' a person and result in the excessive proliferation of hormone-sensitive tissue, thus increasing the risk of hormone-related cancers. Their effect is not, however, quite so straightforward as this explanation suggests. These chemicals basically mess up the hormonal messages the body sends out, changing sexual and reproductive development. They are best thought of as hormone disrupters, interfering with the body's ability to adapt and respond to the environment.

Increased worldwide exposure to these hormone disrupters causes even more concern in light of the findings that a very small change in hormone exposure while the foetus is developing in the womb sets a clock ticking for infertility and increased cancer risk in adulthood. In other words, these chemicals are programming us for extinction. (See Chapter 20 for a more detailed discussion on the issue of declining fertility.)

Another troubling sign is that girls appear to be reaching puberty earlier. The first signs of sexual maturity are now frequently showing at the age of nine, according to US studies. In Britain, the onset of puberty now occurs more often at the age of ten or eleven, compared to thirteen in the 1970s. According to Professor Richard Sharpe of the Medical Research Council, 'If you expose animals to low levels of extra oestrogen neo-natally, they will have advanced puberty.'

Anti-adaptogens

Another way of looking at these chemicals and the broad spectrum of ill effects they appear to be generating is as 'anti-adaptogens'. In other words, they interfere with our innate ability to adapt to the environment – they are a spanner in the works of the neuro-endo-immune network that continuously ensures we adapt our body systems to maintain good health. Coupled with a poor intake of 'adaptogens' – vitamins, minerals, essential fats and phytonutrients – which help to detoxify the body, balance hormones and increase our adaptive potential, these chemicals are leading us towards disaster in terms of ever-decreasing health.

Such substances are thought to disrupt the body's biochemistry because of their ability to lock on to hormone receptor sites. This alters the ability of genes to communicate with the body's cells (known as gene expression), which is vital for good health. In some cases these chemicals actually block a hormone receptor, in other cases they act as if they were the hormone, while some simply disrupt the hormone message. If you think of this 'hormone–hormone receptor–gene expression–biochemical response' sequence as 'communication', what these chemicals do is turn the sound up or down and scramble the message. This is because they don't fit the receptor site perfectly. Human chemistry hasn't been exposed to them throughout our evolution and hasn't managed to adapt its response to deal with them.

The Trouble with Synthetic Hormones

The same is true of synthetic hormones. Take progesterone, for example. When naturally produced by the body it has a precise chemical structure: only this exact molecule can trigger a precise set of instructions to maintain pregnancy, bone density, normal menstruation and other aspects of the hormonal dance that occurs in every woman. It has, even at levels considerably higher than those produced by the human body, remarkably little toxicity.

Yet, almost without exception, every contraceptive pill or HRT prescription, be it a pill, patch or depot, contains synthetic progestins – molecules that are similar to but different from genuine progesterone. They are like keys that will open a lock but don't fit exactly, and so they generate a wobble in the biochemistry of the body. Not surprisingly, the body becomes more toxic; some of the side-effects are increased risk of diseases such as breast cancer, against which the natural molecule is actually protective.

The same applies to oestrogen, or more correctly oestrogens, a family of which is produced naturally. The main three are oestriol, oestrone and oestradiol. During pregnancy oestriol is produced in significantly larger quantities than at other times, when oestrone and oestradiol predominate. Many pharmaceutical drugs, including contraceptive pills and HRT, use synthetic oestrogens which mimic the effects of these naturally occurring molecules.

There could be no more dramatic example of the danger of altering our exposure to these powerful hormone-mimickers than DES, the first synthetic oestrogen, created by Dr Charles Dodds in 1938. Within twenty years, DES was being given to women and to animals. For the latter it improved growth rates, while for women it apparently promised a trouble-free pregnancy and healthier offspring. Eventually, up to 6 million mothers and babies were exposed to DES. It wasn't until 1970 that the flaws surfaced. Girls whose mothers had been on DES during pregnancy started to show abnormalities in their genital development and a substantial increase in cancer rates, especially vaginal cancer of a kind never seen before.[47] Then it was discovered that boys of mothers who had taken DES also had defects in the development of their sexual organs.[48] Many DES children died and many more were infertile.

The danger of synthetic hormones lies not just in the subtle differences in their chemical structure and effect, but also in the amounts given and the balance with other hormones. The amounts of hormones in a contraceptive pill or HRT treatment can be many times higher than the body would produce naturally. Oestrogen produced by the body is balanced with progesterone, but if this balance is lost a health problem is created.

Unopposed oestrogen linked to cancer

Excessive exposure to oestrogen and oestrogen-mimickers may be a major factor behind hormone-related cancers. If breast cells are exposed to oestrogen, their rate of abnormal proliferation doubles.[49] A study by Dr Bergkvist and colleagues in Scandinavia showed that if a woman is on HRT for longer than five years she doubles her risk of breast cancer.[50] They also found that if the HRT included progestins, the synthetic 'cousin' of natural progesterone, that risk was even higher. A large-scale study published in the *New England Journal of Medicine* in 1995 showed that post-menopausal women who had been on HRT for five or more years have a 71 per cent increased risk of breast cancer.[51] The risk was found to increase the longer a woman was on HRT. Overall, there was a 32 per cent increased risk among women using oestrogen HRT, and a 41 per cent risk for those using oestrogen and synthetic progestin HRT, compared to women who had never been on HRT. Another study published in 1995 was carried out by the Emery University School for Public Health: the researchers followed 240,000 women for eight years and found that the risk of ovarian cancer was 72 per cent higher in women given oestrogen HRT.[52] All these studies found that long-term HRT with oestrogen and/or synthetic progestins increased breast cancer risk.

Dr John Lee, from California, a medical expert in female hormones and health, believes that

> The major cause of breast cancer is unopposed oestrogen and there are many factors that would lead to this. Stress, for example, raises cortisol and competes with progesterone for receptor sites. Xenoestrogens from the environment have the ability to damage tissue and lead to an increased risk of cancer later in life. There are also clearly nutritional and genetic factors to consider. What is most concerning is that doctors continue to prescribe unopposed oestrogen to women.

Dietary oestrogens

Natural oestrogens also come to us from food. Meat contains significant amounts of oestrogen, as does dairy produce, although the high levels in these foods may indicate why they aren't perhaps as natural as we would like to think. Much of the meat we eat comes from animals whose feed contains hormones. This, coupled with a high protein intake, speeds up the growth of the animal, which means more profit. Changes in farming practices now make it possible to milk cows continuously, even while pregnant. During pregnancy, oestrogen concentrations in milk go up. While calves may benefit from this extra oestrogen, we do not.

Meat and dairy products are also a storage site for non-degradable toxins which accumulate along the food chain. Millions of tons of chemicals, like non-biodegradable PCBs and DDT, have been released into the environment. Livestock, fish and fowl variously feed on other animals or on pastures or water contaminated with these non-degradable chemicals. Traces accumulate in fat, and when we eat fat in, say, lamb or chicken or milk the chemicals accumulate in us.

Plants too contain natural, oestrogen-like compounds, known as phyto-oestrogens. These are found in a wide variety of foods including soya, citrus fruits, wheat, licorice, alfalfa, celery and fennel. The richest source is soya and its by-products such as tofu or soya milk. However, unlike oestrogenic chemicals such as PCBs, these phyto-oestrogens are associated with a reduced risk of cancer. A high dietary intake of isoflavones, the active ingredient in soya, is associated with a halving of breast cancer in animals, and a substantial reduction in deaths from prostate cancer in men.[53,54] Even more encouraging are animal studies which show that eating a small amount of isoflavones in early infancy results in a 60 per cent reduced risk of breast cancer later in life.[55]

There is no clear explanation of this anomaly, although two theories do exist. One is that these naturally occurring phyto-oestrogens may act as adaptogens and help the body to stabilise hormone levels. The other is that they may block the action of other more toxic environmental oestrogens, perhaps by occupying the receptor sites.

While consuming phyto-oestrogens appears to have positive effects in adults, there is concern about very high intakes during the critical early years of development, such as bottle-feeding an infant a soya-based formula. No one knows yet if this is potentially beneficial or detrimental for hormonal health later in life.

Avoiding the Hormone Disrupters

Why, you may ask, don't we just ban all these hormone-disrupting chemicals? Professor Louis Guillette from the University of Florida asks, 'Should we change policy? Should we be upset? I think we should be fundamentally upset. I think we should be screaming in the streets.' Yet, the reality, until large-scale government action is taken, is that it isn't easy to eliminate all these substances because they are all around us, in our food, water, air and household products. Remember, until the plastics industry either stops using all suspect chemicals, or discloses which chemicals are contained in their products, you have no way of knowing if hormone–disrupting chemicals are present or not. There are, however, steps you can take to make substantial reductions in your own and your family's exposure:

- **Eat organic.** This instantly minimises your exposure to pesticides and herbicides. When you are eating non-organic produce add 2 tablespoons of vinegar to your bowl of washing water. This will reduce pesticides.

- **Filter all drinking water.** I recommend getting a water filter that you install under the sink, made from stainless steel (not plastic or aluminium) and employing a carbon-filtration system. Jug filters work, but generally not as well, depending on how often you change the filter. While not proven to remove all hormone-disrupting chemicals, this should decrease your load. The alternative is spring water, preferably bottled in glass.

- **Reduce your intake of fatty foods.** As explained above, non-biodegradable chemicals accumulate in the food chain in animal fat. Minimising your intake of animal fat – meat and dairy produce – lessens your exposure. There is no need to limit essential fats in nuts and seeds.

- **Never heat food in plastic.** This means goodbye to microwaved TV dinners. If you have to eat this kind of food, transfer the food into a glass container before heating it.

- **Minimise fatty foods in plastic.** Some chemicals that keep plastics flexible easily pass out of the plastic into fatty food – crisps, cheeses, butter, chocolate and pies etc.

- **Minimise liquid foods in soft plastic.** This not only includes fruit juices in cardboard packs, which have a plastic inner lining, but also some fruits and vegetables in cans, which may again have a plastic inner lining.

- **Minimise exposure of food to soft plastic.** This means buying your fruit and vegetables in paper bags rather than in plastic trays covered with cling-film.

- **Switch to natural detergents.** For washing up, washing clothes and personal hygiene use only ecological detergent products from companies who declare all their ingredients. Also, rinse dishes and cutlery after washing up.

- **Don't use pesticides in your garden.** Some pesticides are hormone disruptors. Unless you're sure a product isn't, it's better not to spray. The incidence of childhood cancer is higher in homes whose gardens are sprayed with pesticides.

TEN

BALANCING HORMONES NATURALLY

Whether due to an overload of xeno–oestrogens (oestrogenic chemicals in the environment), synthetic oestrogen in the Pill, HRT or dietary sources (principally meat and dairy produce), more and more women are suffering from what is known as oestrogen dominance – a higher-than-normal ratio of oestrogen to progesterone. Signs of this include:

- PMS
- breast cancer
- weight gain
- ovarian cysts
- menopausal problems
- endometriosis
- breast lumps
- osteoporosis
- fibroids
- infertility

The first step to take, in the presence of any one of these factors, is to cut down your exposure to oestrogen and pursue a nutritional and lifestyle strategy aimed at helping the body to balance hormone levels.

Decrease stress, sugar and stimulants

Stress, or the regular consumption of sugar and stimulants, raises levels of the adrenal hormone cortisol (see Chapter 16). This hormone competes with progesterone and can, therefore, further increase oestrogen dominance.

Decrease your intake of meat and dairy produce

These sources of saturated fats and oestrogenic hormones are best kept to a minimum. If you do eat meat, make sure it's free-range or organic.

Increase dietary intake of essential fats

The body's response to hormones is also controlled by prostaglandins, substances derived from essential fats in the diet. This is why evening primrose oil has proved successful in alleviating symptoms of pre-menstrual syndrome (PMS). The best dietary sources of essential fats are seeds and fish. Sesame and sunflower seeds are high in one type, called omega-6, while flax seeds, pumpkin seeds and carnivorous fish, such as salmon, tuna, herring and mackerel, are rich in the other type, omega-3. We need the equivalent of a heaped tablespoon of these combined seeds a day, or a tablespoon of their oil.

Supplement essential fats

One way to help rapidly restore your hormone balance is to supplement more potent sources of essential fats. These are needed by the immune, nervous and endocrine systems, and are frequently deficient in today's diet. Evening prim-rose oil and borage (starflower) oil contain a potent essential fat called gamma-linolenic acid (GLA) which, supplemented at a level of 150–300mg a day, helps to balance hormones and alleviate symptoms of PMS.[56]

Increase vitamin B6, magnesium and zinc

Many vitamins and minerals are involved in maintaining hormone balance in the body. For this reason it is sensible to supplement a good, all-round multivitamin and mineral. But beyond this there are three nutrients that have repeatedly been shown to help alleviate hormone problems. These are vitamin B6 (100–200mg a day), magnesium (200–400mg a day) and zinc (20mg a day). One recent study at the Institute for Optimum Nutrition, involving 182 women, found that supplementing B6 and magnesium was twice as effective as B6 alone.[57] Vitamin B6 cannot work without adequate zinc, which also has numerous roles to play in balancing hormones, as well as being critical for fertility. These nutrients, plus essential fats, are the 'adaptogens' of your hormone system.

Check your hormone levels

Tremendous advances have been made in testing hormone levels. It is now generally considered that measuring levels of hormones in saliva may be at least as accurate as, if not better than, testing blood levels. A number of laboratories offer simple saliva tests to determine your balance of oestrogen (oestradiol) and progesterone. If you have hormone-related problems ask your nutrition consultant or doctor about these tests.

Consider supplementing natural progesterone

If testing shows you have oestrogen dominance you may benefit from natural progesterone. This is the identical molecule that the body produces and, if given in normal physiological amounts (in other words, equivalent only to what the body produces) can help restore hormone balance.

Natural progesterone: the forgotten hormone

While there are clear reasons for concern about taking in extra oestrogen or synthetic progestins, natural progesterone – identical to that produced in the body – presents a different story. Even at levels several times higher than those produced by the body, it has no known toxicity and has offered no evidence of increased risk of disease. In fact, exactly the opposite has shown to be the case. If breast cancer cells are exposed to progesterone at normal physiological levels, multiplication of cells decreases dramatically.[49] While oestrogen promotes the proliferation of breast cancers, progesterone is protective. A twenty-year study by Dr Mohr, from the Imperial Cancer Research fund at Guy's Hospital, London, showed that women with breast cancer who were treated with natural progesterone had twice the survival rates of those who were not.[58] According to Dr John Lee, author of *Natural Progesterone*, 'Since 1978, I have treated many women with a diagnosis of breast cancer. Not one has had a recurrence. Of the thousands of women using progesterone for other reasons not one has called to say they have breast cancer following use of the natural progesterone cream. It is completely safe and beneficial to give to women with breast cancer.'

Fertility rights

To understand why progesterone is so important it's necessary to understand its role in the menstrual cycle, shown in the diagram overleaf. In the first part of the menstrual cycle, after menstruation, oestrogen levels rise. This stimulates the eggs (ova) in the ovary to grow. It also prepares the endometrial tissue lining the womb to receive a fertilised egg. In other words, oestrogen makes things grow. At the point of ovulation, when one egg is fully matured and released, oestrogen levels reach a peak and then fall. Provided the egg is released, the sac in which the egg matured, called the corpus luteum, starts to produce increasing amounts of progesterone. If the egg is not fertilised, both oestrogen and progesterone levels then fall, stimulating menstruation.

If the egg is fertilised, pregnancy will only be sustained if progesterone levels stay high. For this to happen, the corpus luteum keeps growing and producing progesterone. Eventually, the placenta takes over and produces its own.

One cause of infertility is inadequate nutrition. In one study at the University of Surrey, infertile couples eliminated from their diet alcohol, refined foods and foods to which tests had shown they were allergic; they also supplemented vitamins and minerals in which tests had found them deficient. After this 81 per cent conceived and went on to give birth to

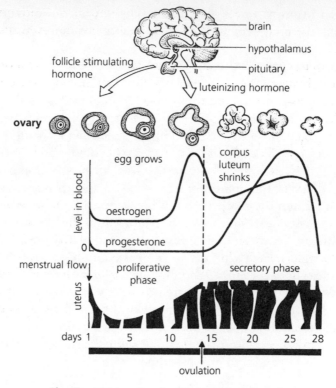

Fig. 5   Hormones in the menstrual cycle

healthy babies. There were no miscarriages, premature births, or children born with deformities.[59] Of course, these vitamins and minerals also help the body make and use hormones, a deficiency of which can result in infertility.

A major cause of miscarriage is a lack of progesterone in the first few weeks after conception. Women with a history of early miscarriage may benefit from progesterone therapy, which involves applying progesterone cream twice a day for absorption through the skin; incidentally, it is also an excellent moisturiser. Only a normal physiological dose is given. The cream is available from your doctor on prescription; in case of difficulty, or for more information, contact the Natural Progesterone Information Service (see p. 210).

Progesterone therapy is also particularly helpful for women who don't always ovulate. In this case it is given only in the last two weeks of the menstrual cycle, when the body would naturally produce progesterone. If a woman doesn't ovulate no progesterone is produced and her oestrogen remains unopposed. Very strenuous exercise is known to suppress ovulation. For example, Dr Peter Ellison from Harvard University tested salivary hormone levels in eighteen regularly cycling, sexually active women with an average age of twenty-nine, and found that seven of them were not ovulating.[60] Even in women who do not take hard exercise, however, anovulatory cycles are exceedingly common.

Leading up to the menopause, a woman starts to have many more anovulatory cycles. Even though her oestrogen levels are decreasing, no ovulation means no progesterone, leading to oestrogen dominance.

The Menopause Connection

The years leading up to the menopause are a prime time to suspect oestrogen dominance. This may be surprising, since we are led to believe that it is the decline in oestrogen that brings on the cessation of menstruation.

All the steps recommended at the beginning of this chapter to keep hormone levels balanced help to reduce menopause symptoms. In fact, many women following nutritional strategies have no menopausal symptoms at all. As one woman told me, at the age of fifty-seven, 'It was a non-event. My energy is good, my mind is sharp.' She lived on a farm, eating organic produce, and took dietary supplements.

However, many women do experience symptoms of the menopause, including:

- hot flushes
- sweats
- mood swings
- insomnia
- headaches
- poor memory
- vaginal dryness

These symptoms sometimes respond to oestrogen HRT, but one in 7 women quit within a year, often due to unpleasant side-effects.

According to Dr John Lee, author of *What Your Doctor Didn't Tell You about the Menopause*, 'The vast majority of menopausal problems can be avoided by good nutrition, avoidance of toxins, regular exercise and the proper supplementation, when indicated for hormonal balance, of natural progesterone.'

The big difference between HRT and natural progesterone treatment is that, while oestrogen and progestins appear to increase the risk of breast cancer, natural progesterone reduces it. What's more, natural progesterone confers significantly greater protection against osteoporosis, as the next chapter explains.

ELEVEN

Osteoporosis – A Skeleton in the Cupboard

Osteoporosis is the silent thief that can rob your skeleton of up to 25 per cent of its bone mass by the time you reach fifty. As a result, one in 3 women, and one in 12 men, have had a fracture by the age of seventy, most commonly of the hip. In the UK fifty thousand people fracture a bone as a result of osteoporosis every year – that's one every three minutes.

Yet osteoporosis is far from inevitable. In fact, in some communities there is no apparent loss of bone density after the menopause. Despite our better diet, analyses of skeletal remains show less bone loss in the eighteenth century than in the late twentieth century. So what has changed? According to a report in the *American Journal of Epidemiology*,[61] an eleven-year-study of forty thousand elderly Norwegians found increased risk of hip fractures among those eating a diet high in non-dairy protein (meat/fish/eggs), or with a high coffee or low calcium intake.

Too Much Protein

One consistent finding is that those who eat a high-protein diet increase their risk of osteoporosis: communities with high protein intakes have high rates of the disease. This is almost certainly because protein-rich foods are acid-forming once inside the body. The body cannot tolerate substantial changes in the acid/alkaline balance of the blood and therefore neutralises or 'buffers' this effect using two main alkaline agents – sodium and calcium. When the body's reserves of sodium are used up, calcium is taken from the bones. Therefore, the more protein you eat the more calcium you need.

The fact that high-protein diets lead to calcium deficiency is nothing new. But research is increasingly showing that, if you eat a high-protein diet, no amount of calcium corrects the imbalance. In one study published in the

American Journal of Clinical Nutrition, some subjects were given a moderately high-protein diet (80g of protein a day) and others a very high-protein diet (240g a day) plus 1400mg of calcium. The overall loss of calcium was 37mg per day on the high-protein diet and 137mg per day on the very high-protein diet.[62] The authors concluded that 'high-calcium diets are unlikely to prevent probable bone loss induced by high-protein diets'. In another study, a protein intake of 95g a day (bacon and eggs for breakfast supplies 55g) resulted in an average calcium loss of 58mg per day, which means a loss of 2 per cent of total skeletal calcium per year – that's 20 per cent each decade.[63] Some medical scientists now believe that a lifelong high-protein, acid-forming diet may be a primary cause of osteoporosis.

Not Enough Calcium?

The obvious conclusion to be drawn from the high protein–calcium loss link is that, if you lose calcium from the bone, taking in more would put it back. Yet it seems that, unless your calcium intake is very low indeed, calcium supplementation alone makes little difference. Calcium balance in the body depends on many factors, and the following can all stop the body making the best use of dietary calcium:

- lack of magnesium
- lack of exercise
- lack of stomach acid
- too much protein
- too much stress
- too much coffee

A person with a relatively low intake of calcium, but none of the above problems, may have better calcium status than someone who is apparently consuming enough calcium but scores high on the factors listed above.

The Hormone Connection

The conventional explanation of osteoporosis is that once a woman stops menstruating she produces less oestrogen, which normally helps keep calcium in the bones. Hence the recommendation for women to have hormone replacement therapy to protect their bones. This is far from the truth, though.

Bones have two kinds of cells: osteoblasts, which build new cells, and osteoclasts, which get rid of old bone material such as calcium. Oestrogen, which stimulates osteoclast cells, only stops the loss of old bone. Progesterone, on the other hand, stimulates osteoblasts which build new bone. Taking natural progesterone increases your bone density four times more than taking oestrogen does.

In the time leading up to the menopause, a woman gradually stops ovu-lating. If no egg is released, no progesterone is produced, even though her body continues to produce small amounts of oestrogen. Scientists are now coming round to thinking that it is the relative excess of oestrogen to progesterone – creating a progesterone deficiency – that is precipitating osteoporosis, rather than the deficiency in oestrogen.

Say No to Osteoporosis

The best way to prevent osteoporosis is to combine all these prevention strategies. This means following all the advice in Chapter 10, plus:

- **Don't consume more than 40g of protein a day.** This is not usually a problem for vegetarians, who should aim to have two servings a day of a high-protein vegetable food such as lentils, beans or tofu. For a meat-eater this means eating meat no more than once a day, and ideally no more than three times a week.

- **Eat fish rather than meat.** Fish is preferable, because it provides more essential fats and fewer oestrogenic hormones.

- **Rely on seeds and nuts for minerals, not on dairy products.** Dairy products, especially cheese, are high in protein and oestrogenic hormones and low in magnesium. Remember, our ancestors didn't milk buffaloes. They got their calcium and other minerals from seeds, nuts and vege-tables. A heaped tablespoon of ground seeds a day gives you plenty of calcium, magnesium and many other essential nutrients.

- **Supplement a bone mineral complex.** This should include a daily 500mg of calcium, 350mg of magnesium, 400ius of vitamin D, 2mg of boron, 10mg of zinc and 1000mg vitamin C.

- **Avoid coffee.** High coffee intake is associated with low bone density.

- **Exercise every other day.** The best kind of exercise is weight-bearing, preferably using both lower and upper body muscles. Even walking for fifteen minutes makes a difference.

- **Use natural progesterone cream.** If you are pre-menopausal have your hormone levels checked and, if you turn out to be oestrogen-dominant, ask your doctor to prescribe natural progesterone. If you are post-menopausal, do this anyway. In case of difficulty, or for information, contact the Natural Progesterone Information Service (see p. 210).

PART 4

THE POWER OF PREVENTION

If the doctors of today don't become the nutritionists of tomorrow, the nutritionists of today will be the doctors of tomorrow.

DR PAAVO AIROLA

TWELVE

HALTING THE CANCER EPIDEMIC

According to a survey by the East Anglian Cancer Intelligence Unit at Cambridge University, we are heading for a cancer epidemic.[44] While cancer is currently the second most common cause of death in the UK and USA, within twenty years the risk of developing cancer at some time during your life will be greater than 50 per cent. Conventional treatment for cancer is all very medieval in concept – cut it out, burn it out or drug it out – and contrary to popular newspaper reports of 'miracle drugs' that are supposedly on the verge of being released, figures show that we are losing the cancer war, not winning it.

Of particular concern is the rise in hormone-related cancers. These are cancers of hormonally sensitive tissue which, in men, are the prostate gland and testes and, in women, the cervix, ovaries, breasts and womb tissue. Take breast cancer, for example. Currently, one in 12 women in the USA develops breast cancer – in the UK one in 8. We are told that, in the last thirty years, the survival rate has increased from 60 to 75 per cent. The death rate from cancer over the same period has stayed the same. All that's happened is that people are being diagnosed earlier, and so appear to survive longer. The incidence of a type of cervical cancer, adenocarcinoma, has also gone up fourfold in twenty years. It is predicted that within twenty years one in 4 men will develop prostate cancer.[44] In truth, these hormone-related cancers are occurring more frequently and earlier in our lives than they did a decade ago. It is highly likely that changes in diet and our exposure to environmental toxins are playing a significant role.

Genes or Environment?

There is little doubt that some people have genetic differences that increase their potential for certain kinds of cancer. There is, for example, a strain of mice which, when exposed to UVB radiation, will develop skin cancer unless they are given supplements of silymarin, an antioxidant found in the herb milk thistle, according to a study published recently in the *Journal of the National Cancer Institute*.[64]

This tells us, firstly, that a genetic predisposition to cancer can only become a reality if you are exposed to certain cancer-causing agents, known as carcinogens – in this case, excessive sunlight. Secondly, it says that even with exposure, if your intake of anti-cancer agents is sufficient you can still prevent its occurrence.

So genes that predispose you to cancer do exist, and are known as 'onco-genes'. Yet they are only activated by the presence of certain carcinogens. Even if you don't have these oncogenes, some carcinogens can damage cells so that they start to behave inappropriately. Alternatively, poor nutrition, for example a lack of the B vitamin folic acid, can result in gene damage; once again, your cells can start to behave abnormally. Some carcinogens don't actually initiate cancer, but promote it once the process has begun. Cancer of the upper digestive tract, the oesophagus, is often triggered by smoking and promoted by drinking alcohol, possibly through its suppression of the immune system.

So there are many factors that must be present to switch a normal cell into a cancer cell. Unlike normal cells, cancer cells start to disrespect their boundaries and invade the space of others. Normally, the immune system will respond by wiping out such misbehaving cells. But if the immune response isn't strong enough, the cancer mass takes over. In due course, the cancer spreads to other parts of the body. This process is known as 'metastasis' and produces secondary tumours. It is these secondaries, not the primary tumour, that are nearly always responsible for death.

With this model in mind, cancer can be seen as a disease process in which the 'self-organising' aspect of the body breaks down. It's as if the cells can no longer adapt to a new set of circumstances. Simply to focus on destroying the tumour is to deny its underlying causes. There are many ways either to prevent cancer or to maximise the chances of a full recovery from it: eliminating carcinogens and substances that trigger cancer by 'reprograming' genes; and increasing your intake of substances that are 'anti-cancer' because they block carcinogens, boost the immune system, or stop the cancer growing and spreading to other parts of the body.

Eliminating Carcinogens

Many common substances to which we are exposed are known carcinogens. Although the level that triggers cancer may be a lot higher than most people are normally exposed to, a cursory look down the checklist overleaf will show that, like most people, you are probably exposed to a large number of potential carcinogens. You may wonder what the cumulative effect of

Carcinogens to Avoid

The following factors are carcinogenic only at certain concentrations. While it is ideal to minimise your overall exposure or intake, the presence of these carcinogens in small amounts may not constitute a risk.

Carcinogens in daily use or commonly occurring
- Tobacco smoke, whether or not you are the smoker.
- Coal tar and petrochemical derivatives used in some hair oils, lipsticks and cosmetics, perfumes, soaps, deodorants and anti-perspirants.
- Plastics containing vinyl chloride, polystyrene, and certain plasticisers e.g. food containers, kitchen utensils, clothes, furniture, curtains, bedding etc.
- Fluoride in water supplies and in toothpaste.
- Epoxy resins, glues etc.
- Carbon tetrachloride (used in cleaning fluids, etc.)
- Many factory emissions, especially containing sulfuric acid.
- Car, lorry, bus and boat exhausts and fumes from central heating boilers (oil, coal or gas fired).
- Food preservatives, especially nitrates in bacon, tinned meat, ham, sausage etc.

Carcinogens and potential carcinogens in food and drink
- Chlorine in tap water.
- Pesticides and their residues.
- Insecticides.
- Smoked meats and fish (such food often contains creosote and formalde-hyde).
- Nitrites are formed from nitrates and combine with amines in the gut to form nitrosamines, these are cancer inducing. Found in processed meats, non-organic fruit and vegetables and water from over-use of nitrogen fertilisers in agriculture.
- Coffee is suspect because, in the roasting, matrol is produced.
- Decaffeinated coffee also contains matrol.
- Saccharin (chemical sweetener).
- Saturated fat (found in dairy produce, meat and meat products, pastry, cakes and puddings, cheese, milk, eggs, fish and chips, and other fried foods).
- Cyclamates (chemical sweetener).
- Fats heated to high temperatures (above 200°C or 392°F in preparing food). Frying is therefore not recommended.
- Alcohol – risk is significant above one drink a day for women and two drinks a day for men.
- Parsley, celery, parsnips, these and other members of the *Umbellifereae* family contain carcinogenic psoralens.

- Burnt (charred or dark brown) foods (e.g. toast, cakes, bread) and charred or brown meat. Cut all dark pieces away.
- Bleaches (for flour, white bread etc.).
- Moulds on foodstuffs such as *Aspergillus flavus* and the toxin aflatoxin, and other mycotoxins found in certain moulds e.g. on nuts, cheese, milk, jam, bread.

Medical carcinogens
- Chloroform.
- Liquid paraffin.
- X-rays (including radioactive dyes and radio isotopes).
- All mineral oil.
- All coal-derivative products.
- Hormone therapy (contraceptive pills and HRT)
- Certain antibiotics and sulphonamide drugs are strongly suspect (certainly they can trigger animal cancers).
- Psoralens (used for treating skin complaints).
- Tamoxifen (the anti-cancer drug).

Other carcinogens
- Background from nuclear radiation which pollutes the atmosphere, crops, meat and water.
- Certain viruses.
- Radiation from TV sets, computers and mobile phones.
- Radiation from the sun.

consuming a number of known carcinogens, albeit at low doses. In truth, no one knows, but the results from the laboratory of Professor Ana Soto and Professor Carlos Sonnenschein at Boston's Tufts University are alarming. They were investigating the levels at which known oestrogenic chemicals (see Chapter 9) would cause proliferation of breast cancer cells. They then exposed these cells to a combination of five or ten chemicals, each at a tenth of the dose that would produce proliferation. Sure enough, there was a cocktail effect: in combination these chemicals were many times as powerful as on their own, producing rapid proliferation of breast cancer cells.[65]

Because we do not fully understand the effect of combinations of mild carcinogens, and because it would take decades to find out, the only sensible way forward is to follow a diet and lifestyle that reduce our exposure to these substances. Where smoking is concerned, the necessary action is clear-cut: don't do it. The same can be said for pesticides: eat organic. However, it is a trickier decision where a number of carcinogenic substances are concerned, such as those found in plastics. As plastics manufacturers aren't at present required to disclose the chemicals in their products, and as not all the substances used have yet been tested, it is probably best not to eat very much food (especially acidic or fatty food) that has been exposed to plastic for more than a day or two (see Chapters 9 and 20).

Beyond Antioxidants

The first major preventive approaches to cancer hinged on the understanding that oxidants, often the by-products of combustion, acted as carcinogens by damaging genes and triggering cancer. These oxidants include cigarette smoke, car exhausts, industrial pollutants and radiation (sunlight or man-made).

The discovery that vitamins A, C and E and, more recently, the mineral selenium, could disarm these oxidants led to investigations into their anti-cancer properties. Results to date have been very impressive, although we are beginning to understand that the role of a number of anti-cancer agents goes deeper than simply disarming carcinogens. Vitamin A, for example, not only controls cell growth but also stimulates communication between them. Isoflavones help to regulate hormone levels and counter the negative effects of excess oestrogen or testosterone, reducing the risk of breast and prostate cancer.

These anti-cancer agents may be best thought of as 'adaptogens', substances that help us to adapt to a hostile environment. They are widely available in nature, which suggests a cooperative evolution between us and our natural environment. Many of today's most significant carcinogens are man-made – the result of not respecting our relationship with the environment. Cancer may be seen as a consequence of too many carcinogens and too few adaptogens, leading to a breakdown in communication. Tilting the equation back the other way is the best way we know at present of preventing or reversing cancer.

Increasing Adaptogens – the Keys to Cancer Prevention

Vitamin A and betacarotene

Both vitamin A and its precursor, betacarotene (which the body can convert into vitamin A) possess anti-cancer properties. People with lung cancer have greatly reduced levels of vitamin A in their blood.[66] Those who eat very little

vitamin A in their diet have twice as high a risk of lung cancer as those people who consume a lot of vitamin A. Similarly, a high intake of betacarotene
from raw fruit and vegetables reduces the risk of lung cancer in non-smoking
men and women,[67] as well as reducing the risk of cancer of the stomach,
colon, prostate and cervix. In one study, supplementing 30mg of betacarotene a day resulted in the improvement of 71 per cent of patients with
oral pre-cancer (leukoplakia), while 200,000iu of vitamin A a week resulted
in 57 per cent of patients having complete remission.[68] The ideal daily intake
of vitamin A is 5000–10,000ius of vitamin A and 15–25mg of betacarotene.

Vitamin C

Although first shown to be a powerful anti-cancer agent in 1971, vitamin C
didn't start to be accepted in this role by the medical profession for another
twenty years. In 1992 Dr Gladys Bock, formerly with the US National
Cancer Institute, wrote, 'I have reviewed the epidemiologic literature, about
140 studies, on the relationship between antioxidant micronutrients or their
food sources and cancer risk. The data are overwhelmingly consistent. With
possibly fewer than five exceptions, every single study is in the protective
direction, and something like 110 to 120 studies found statistically significant
reduced risk with high intake.' Vitamin C-rich diets reduce the risk of
cancer, and high intakes – above 5000mg a day (the equivalent of 100
oranges) – substantially increase the life expectancy of cancer patients.

In the first-ever study, by Dr Linus Pauling and Dr Ewan Cameron in the
1970s, 100 terminally ill cancer patients were given 10g (10,000mg) of
vitamin C each day and their outcome compared with that of 1000 cancer
patients given conventional therapy. The survival rate was five times higher
in those taking vitamin C and by 1978, while all the 1000 'control patients'
had died, 13 of the vitamin C patients were still alive, with 12 apparently free
from cancer.[69] More recent studies have confirmed these findings. Dr Murata
and Dr Morishige of Saga University in Japan showed that cancer patients on
5–30g of vitamin C a day lived six times longer than those on 4g or less, while
those suffering from cancer of the uterus lived fifteen times longer on vitamin C therapy.[70] These studies show that, while 1–5g of vitamin C may prevent cancer, cancer patients benefit most from 10g or more a day.

Vitamin E

While vitamin C is a water-based antioxidant, protecting the watery parts of
the body, vitamin E is a fat-based antioxidant and protects cell membranes
and structural fats. The two work together, helping to increase each other's
effectiveness. Research in 1984 in Britain, led by Dr Wald at St Bartholo-
mew's Hospital in London, found that 'those with the lowest vitamin E levels

have the highest risk of breast cancer.[71] Another study measured blood levels of vitamin E and selenium; those in the top third had a 91 per cent decreased risk of cancer. The findings of the most recent trial to date, involving 2569 women with breast cancer, concluded that 'a diet rich in several micro-nutrients, especially betacarotene, vitamin E and calcium, may be protective against breast cancer.[72] These are but a few examples from a wealth of data that links breast cancer with low vitamin E levels, and prevention of breast cancer with increased vitamin E intake. An optimal intake of breast cancer prevention is between 400 and 800ius/mg per day.

Selenium

Vitamin E also works hand-in-hand with the mineral selenium. In the work of Dr Jukka Salonen and colleagues in Finland blood samples were taken from 12,155 people. Four years later 51 had died of cancer; those with both low vitamin E and selenium had eleven times the risk of death from cancer and those with adequate levels.[73] A recent trial by Dr Larry Clark and colleagues at Cornell University in the USA gave one group of people 200mcg of selenium and another group a placebo. The researchers found a significant reduction in the incidence of lung, colorectal and prostate cancer, and reduced mortality from lung cancer, amongst the selenium group.[74] These studies are just a small sample from over four hundred studies which indicate that selenium plays a role in cancer prevention. The ideal intake is between 100 and 200mcg daily, though the average diet provides no more than 50mcg. Selenium is found in large quantities in fish and seeds.

Other antioxidants

While those listed above are the best-known and most researched antioxidants, they are by no means the only highly protective ones. Other antioxidants known to be cancer-protective include silymarin from the herb milk thistle, proanthocyanidins from berries and fruits, glutathione and cysteine, which is plentiful in garlic. A US National Cancer Institute study carried out in China in 1989 found that those provinces which used garlic liberally had the lowest rate of stomach cancer.

Foods That Fight Cancer

Antioxidant fruit and vegetables

Rich sources of vitamins A and C, these are top of the anti-cancer foods. A study in Japan of 265,000 people found that those with a low intake of betacarotene, which is found in fruits and vegetables, had a higher risk of lung cancer.[75] Other studies have shown similar results for colon, stomach, prostate and cervical cancer. A tomato a day, rich in both betacarotene and lycopene, cuts the risk of pancreatic cancer.[76] Betacarotene is found in particularly high quantities in carrots, broccoli, sweet potatoes, cantaloupe melons and apricots. Vitamin C is abundant in fresh vegetables and fruit. Cruciferous vegetables, which include broccoli, cabbage, cauliflower, Brussels sprouts, turnips, horseradish, kale, kohlrabi, mustard and cress, halve your

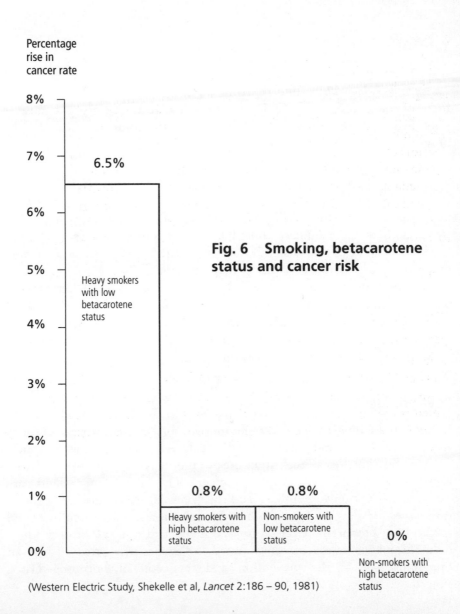

Percentage rise in cancer rate

6.5% — Heavy smokers with low betacarotene status

Fig. 6 Smoking, betacarotene status and cancer risk

0.8% — Heavy smokers with high betacarotene status

0.8% — Non-smokers with low betacarotene status

0% — Non-smokers with high betacarotene status

(Western Electric Study, Shekelle et al, *Lancet* 2:186 – 90, 1981)

risk of colon cancer if eaten three times a week.[78] Eating antioxidant-rich foods has as great an effect in reducing your cancer risk as not smoking.[77]

Fibre

Colon cancer risk can be significantly reduced by including fibre sources such as vegetables, fruit, grains, beans and lentils in your diet. Fibre speeds up the passage of food through the digestive tract and minimises the formation of carcinogens in the bowel.

Yoghurt

It is possible that yoghurt too protects against colon cancer. The bacterium *Lactobacillus acidophilus*, found in many yoghurts, slows down the development of colon tumours, according to research at Tufts University in Boston published in 1990.[83] Abnormal cell divisions in the colon also slowed right down when calcium intake was increased to 2000mg a day.

Fish and fish oils

Supplements of the fish oil EPA (an omega-3 fat) have proved very protective against cancer in animals with a high risk of getting the disease. A daily supplement of 5g of these fish oils can regulate gene expression and increase the production of nitric oxide, which immune cells use to kill cancer cells.[80,81] Fish oils, which are richest in salmon, shark, mackerel, herring and tuna, calm inflammation, which is associated with reduction of the risk of cancer spreading to other parts of the body. Communities which consume a large amount of omega-3 fats in their diet, either from fish or from seeds (especially flax seed), have a low risk of cancer.

Soya products

In Japan and China, women who get most of their protein from soya foods – tofu, soya beans and soya milk – have lower rates of breast cancer, a finding confirmed in animal studies. Soya products are good for men too, lowering their risk of prostate cancer. The active ingredients are isoflavones, including genistein and diadzein. A daily intake of these isoflavones prevents the testosterone excess that is associated with increased risk to both prostate hyperplasia (enlargement) and cancer.[81] Soya produce or the supplementation of concentrated isoflavones may prove to play an important part in the prevention and remission of hormone-related cancers.

Foods to Avoid

Milk can contain significant levels of hormones, as can the meat of animals given growth hormones. Eating a lot of dairy products and meat is associated in particular with cancer of the colon. Other cancer-promoting factors are a high intake of saturated fat, and eating fried or burnt foods which increase the oxidant load on the body. Excess caffeine brings a slightly greater risk of cancer of the bladder,[82] while alcohol increases the possibility of breast, colon and rectal cancers.[83] Alcohol's suppressive effect on the immune system means a greater risk of any cancer spreading. It is most strongly linked to cancers of the oesophagus, lung and stomach.

Why Sharks Don't Get Cancer

Once a cancer mass is formed it develops its own blood supply and defence system. This process is called angiogenesis. It then becomes increasingly difficult for the immune system to deal with the tumour, which now has a life of its own. One strategy, known as anti-angiogenesis, involves cutting off the tumour's blood supply so that the tumour effectively starves to death. In 1976 Dr Robert Langer, of the Massachusetts Institute of Technology, discovered an inhibitor of new blood vessels in tumours – shark cartilage. As cartilage has no blood supply it makes sense that it would contain such an inhibitor. While different kinds of cartilage have been shown to have anti-tumour properties, shark cartilage has proved the most effective to date. This may also explain why the incidence of cancer in sharks, which have no bones, is less than 1 per cent of that of other fish.

Unlike nutritional strategies, which have been tested principally for preventing cancer, shark cartilage has been tested for inducing the remission of advanced cancer. Leading its research is Dr William Lane, author of *Sharks Don't Get Cancer*. To date, trials have been small, but positive.[84] In eight breast cancer cases where the tumours were as large as golfballs, all the women were virtually tumour-free after eleven weeks of taking shark cartilage. In another study by a New Jersey doctor, 76 cancer patients all responded well to shark cartilage. Many studies are now under way and the results are awaited with interest. For maximum effectiveness shark cartilage must be used in high doses, ranging from 60g per day for solid tumours to 15g a day for follow-up prevention.

The Synergy Effect

Dr Richard Passwater, who was the first scientist to discover that vitamins C and E help each other to work, believes that the synergistic effect of increasing one's intake of these 'adaptogens', including antioxidant vitamins and minerals, through diets and supplementation, coupled with a conscious reduction of exposure to carcinogens, can put a halt to the current cancer epidemic and reduce your risk by as much as 70 per cent. This is because the power of synergy (nutrients working together) is far greater than the sum total of the effect of each nutrient in isolation.

In addition to the recommendations given in this chapter, anything you can do to keep the immune system strong is a big plus in preventing cancer. This subject is discussed fully in Chapter 15.

THIRTEEN

A NEW THEORY ON HEART DISEASE

Recent discoveries in science, the environment, evolution and genetics are beginning to unravel the mystery of how we have evolved as a species. Many diseases which we label as bad news may have developed to protect us. When your nose blocks up on exposure to a pollutant, or when the cells in a smoker's lungs change form after repeated exposure to poisons in a cigarette, the body is trying to adapt to new conditions. It is this very ability to adapt that keeps us alive in an ever-changing world.

At the age of ninety-two Dr Linus Pauling proposed that the development of cardiovascular disease, the number one killer in the Western world, may have prevented our extinction. His paper 'A Unified Theory of Human Cardiovascular Disease', co-authored by Dr Matthias Rath, has attracted considerable interest among leading cardiologists.[85] If proved right, this theory will not only solve the riddle of the origin of heart disease, but may lead to its abolition as a cause of human death. The solution? Vitamin C.

All animals except guinea pigs, fruit-eating bats, the red-vented bulbul bird and primates, including man, make vitamin C in their bodies. The amount varies from species to species, but is usually the equivalent of 1000–20,000mg a day in humans. A goat, for example, produces 216mg of vitamin C per kg of body weight. Therefore an adult goat weighing 60kg produces 13,000mg of vitamin C. Yet most people in the Western world currently consume below 100mg – obviously far less than we need. It was about 40 million years ago that man's ancestors lost their ability to synthesise vitamin C from glucose in their bodies, since when we have had to depend on our diet to supply this essential vitamin. The precondition for such a genetic mutation was most likely a plentiful supply in early man's diet. Indeed, it was rich in fruit and other plant material and could easily have provided several grams of vitamin C per day. When our ancestors left tropical regions, however, to settle in other parts of the world (especially during the Ice Ages, when vegetation was very scarce) they would have been at high risk of developing scurvy.

Scurvy is a fatal disease characterised by a breakdown of the connective tissue. Vitamin C is essential for the production of collagen and elastin, which hold all skin, membranes and cells together. The first sign of scurvy is internal bleeding and bruising, as blood vessels start to leak. In earlier centuries blood loss from scurvy decimated ships' crews who could not take fresh fruit and vegetables on long voyages.

Nature on the Defensive

So how did we survive? According to Linus Pauling we may have developed the ability to deposit lipids (fats) and lipoproteins (fat-protein complexes) along the artery walls to protect them, in order to increase our chances of surviving during vitamin C-deficient times. Another group of proteins that normally accumulate at injury sites to effect repair are fibrinogen and apoprotein. The combination of lipoprotein with apoprotein is now thought to be the major genetic development that combated the damaging effects of scurvy on artery walls. These two substances combined are known as lipoprotein A, which, in excess, is now thought to be one of the greatest predictors of developing cardiovascular disease. So now let's look at what is known about the development of atherosclerosis, the thickening and eventual blockage or rupturing of blood vessels that causes strokes, heart attacks, angina and thrombosis.

Cholesterol Revisited

The first theory was that cholesterol, a fat-like substance made by the body, was the culprit. The answer was to cut out dietary cholesterol, but this alone has shown little effect. It was then discovered that it wasn't cholesterol itself that was the problem but how well you could clear it from your arteries. Cholesterol is made in the liver, and should return there once it has been released in bile into the digestive tract, where it helps digest fats and is then absorbed into the bloodstream. Certain protein carriers, known as low-density lipoproteins (LDLs), were found to be responsible for carrying it to the artery wall, and others, high-density lipoproteins (HDLs), were responsible for carrying it through the artery walls and back to the liver. So if you have a low LDL cholesterol count and a high HDL cholesterol count, that would be good news.

Another avenue of thought focussed on the 'fat theory'. Fats in the blood are called triglycerides. These too, if raised, herald heart disease. Unlike the situation with cholesterol, eating too much fat (or sugar or alcohol) does raise blood triglyceride levels.

Recent research is now questioning even this HDL/LDL model. First of all, it appears that oxidised (damaged) cholesterol, whatever kind of lipoprotein it's on, is more prone to clogging up arteries. Normally, cholesterol is protected from oxidation by antioxidant nutrients such as vitamins A, C and E. This fits well with current research, which consistently shows a low risk of atherosclerosis among people with high intakes of antioxidant nutrients. More recent findings are that the 'problem' fat may in fact be lipoprotein A – Lp(a) – a particular combination of fat and protein which transports cholesterol and binds with blood clots. Lipoprotein A can repair damaged or leaky blood vessels, but it also increases the risk of heart disease by building

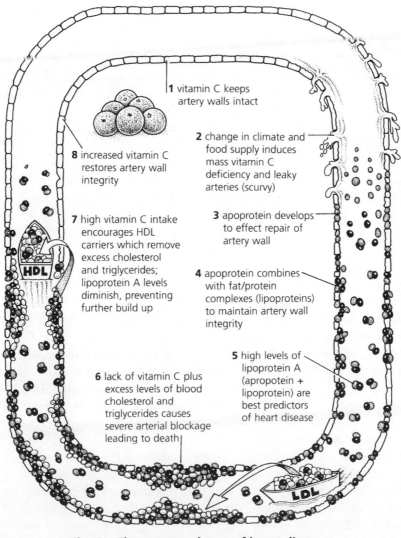

1 vitamin C keeps artery walls intact

8 increased vitamin C restores artery wall integrity

2 change in climate and food supply induces mass vitamin C deficiency and leaky arteries (scurvy)

7 high vitamin C intake encourages HDL carriers which remove excess cholesterol and triglycerides; lipoprotein A levels diminish, preventing further build up

3 apoprotein develops to effect repair of artery wall

4 apoprotein combines with fat/protein complexes (lipoproteins) to maintain artery wall integrity

HDL

6 lack of vitamin C plus excess levels of blood cholesterol and triglycerides causes severe arterial blockage leading to death

5 high levels of lipoprotein A (apropotein + lipoprotein) are best predictors of heart disease

LDL

Fig. 7   The cause and cure of heart disease

up deposits on artery walls. Research is now strongly suggesting that the development of lipoprotein A was most likely a genetic response to a species threatened with extinction because of leaky blood vessels. Could this have been nature's response to life-threatening scurvy? The estimated period of the development of lipoprotein A in monkeys correlates with the time at which primates are thought to have lost the ability to produce vitamin C.

How well does the theory of vitamin C deficiency as a root cause for cardiovascular disease fit with the facts? Vitamin C deficiency raises blood levels of cholesterol, triglycerides, the 'bad' LDLs, apoprotein and Lp(a), and lowers the beneficial HDLs. Conversely, increasing vitamin C intake lowers high cholesterol, triglyceride, LDL or Lp(a) levels and raises HDLs. The chance of all these effects not being a coincidence was too great and led Linus Pauling and his colleagues to investigate further.

The significance of all these beneficial effects for our ancestors, could be that, during the summer months when vitamin C intake was sufficient, the increased HDL production would remove excess cholesterol. Vitamin C also inhibits excessive cholesterol production and stimulates 7-a-hydroxylase, a key enzyme for converting cholesterol to bile. All this would lead to a decrease in unnecessary atherosclerotic deposits. In one study it was shown that 500mg of vitamin C a day can lead to a reduction in atherosclerotic deposits within two to six months. 'This concept also explains why heart attack and stroke occur today with a much higher frequency in winter than spring and summer, the seasons with increased ascorbate intake,' says Pauling.

Genetic Evidence

There is strong evidence that some people have a genetic tendency to develop high cholesterol or high triglycerides or both. According to Pauling's theory, a lack of vitamin C unmasks this tendency, which developed to protect arteries from scurvy.

Two other genetically based cardiovascular diseases are diabetic angiopathy, and homocysteinuria. In diabetes, the very high levels of glucose in the blood interfere with vitamin C intake and exacerbate arterial degeneration. Supplementing vitamin C not only helps to prevent these problems by increasing its concentration in the artery walls but also improves blood glucose and insulin balance.

In homocysteinuria the sufferer accumulates too much of a toxic substance called homocysteine. It is formed from methionine as it is converted to cystanthionine, a harmless substance, but in certain people excess homocysteine accumulates due to an enzyme defect. The result is widespread damage in the cardiovascular system – 60 per cent of patients show clear symptoms before the age of forty. Once again, vitamin C supplementation can prevent these problems and other complications caused by the disease by helping to metabolise homocysteine properly, a difficulty experienced by as many as one in 5 people. Having a raised homocysteine level doubles the risk of a heart attack. The B vitamins, folic acid, B6 and B12 are now known to prevent homocysteine formation and hence reduce risk.

Reversing Atherosclerosis

Of course, the proof of any theory lies in whether or not it works. Treatment for atherosclerosis involves the supplementation of both vitamin C and the amino acid lysine, which together help not only to prevent lipoprotein A from binding to arterial walls, but also to 'undo' arterial deposits. No clinical trials to test this theory have yet been completed, but an increasing number of success stories are being reported.

One such case is of a leading US biochemist who had had three coronary bypass operations, numerous complications and angina (heart pain) at the slightest exertion. He took a lot of medications, including beta-blockers and aspirin, every day. To this medication his cardiologist, who confirmed that a fourth coronary bypass operation was not possible, advised him to add 6g of ascorbic acid (vitamin C) and 60mg of Co-Q10, a multivitamin tablet with minerals, additional vitamins A, E and B complex, lecithin and niacin (B3). Linus Pauling recommended him to continue the ascorbic acid and add 5g of l-lysine daily.

The biochemist started with a daily 1g of lysine in May 1991, and increased the dose to 5g by mid-June. By mid-July he could walk two miles and do gardening without angina pain and wrote, 'The effects of the lysine borders on the miraculous.' He attributed his newfound wellbeing to the addition of lysine and vitamins to his other medications. His wife and friends commented on his renewed vigour.

Michael, a patient of mine who had had three strokes and had suffered from high blood pressure for ten years came to me suffering from angina due to a totally blocked coronary artery. Even a brisk walk gave him extreme chest pain. I prescribed a daily 5g of vitamin C and 3g of lysine, plus 600ius of vitamin E and 30mg of Co-Q 10. Five months later, having stopped taking two drugs for high blood pressure, his blood pressure was normal and he could raise his exercising pulse rate to 180 beats per minute before experiencing any pain.

A Radical Rethink on Heart Disease

Pauling's theory on the cause and treatment of heart disease certainly fits the facts at hand but will inevitably need to be thoroughly tested, in predicting, treating and preventing cardiovascular disease, before it will be widely accepted. If proved right, however, it will necessitate a radical rethink by all those scientists who have pursued other models such as the cholesterol theory. According to the famous German physicist Max Planck, 'An important innovation rarely makes its way by gradually winning over and converting its opponents. What does happen is that its opponents gradually die out and that the growing generation is familiar with the idea from the beginning.' The vitamin C theory may be just such an idea.

Pauling, who died in 1994 at the age of ninety-three, was certainly convinced: 'Cardiovascular disease is the direct consequence of the inability of man to synthesise ascorbate in combination with insufficient intake of ascorbate in the modern diet.' If vitamin C deficiency does prove to be the common cause of human cardiovascular disease, then its supplementation is destined to become the universal treatment. He recommends 5–20g a day. The available epidemiological and clinical evidence is reasonably convincing. In Pauling's words, 'Further clinical confirmation of this theory should lead to the abolition of cardiovascular disease as a cause of human mortality for the present generation and future generations of mankind.'

Minerals and High Blood Pressure

While Pauling and Rath's theory may explain the origin of atherosclerosis and the human predisposition for it, there are unquestionably other factors that contribute to heart and artery disease. One of these is blood pressure control by calcium, magnesium, sodium and potassium. Surrounding the inner wall of arteries is a layer of muscle. This muscle wall can be relaxed or contracted; when it contracts, blood pressure increases. This is a normal response to stress, as it helps get glucose out of the blood and into cells. If, however, this response is prolonged or if the blood vessel concerned is already partially blocked, the result can be high blood pressure or even total blockage, triggering a heart attack or stroke. This state of arterial tension is controlled by the electrical difference of what are known as 'electrolytic' minerals inside and outside the muscle cells.

The minerals in question are calcium, magnesium and potassium, all of which relax the artery, and sodium which contracts it. If each of these first three are given in isolation, they significantly lower blood pressure, while avoiding sodium has the same effect.[86] The effect of each mineral individually is less than that of the common blood pressure-lowering drugs, yet an increase in calcium, magnesium and potassium intake, coupled with a decrease in sodium, can dramatically lower blood pressure within days – equivalent to or better than the drugs, but without the side-effects.[87]

Sodium is easily avoided by not adding salt to food and not eating foods that already contain salt. The best sources of calcium and magnesium are seeds (sesame and sunflower) and nuts (almonds), while there is lots of potassium in fruit. (Dairy products, although high in calcium, are a poor source of magnesium.) Of the three, magnesium is the most commonly deficient and it's well worth supplementing 500mg of both calcium and magnesium if you have high blood pressure. Magnesium also helps the heart to function; optimal levels are strongly related to decreasing risk for heart disease.[88]

Protect Your Cholesterol

Cholesterol, like any fatty substance, is prone to oxidant damage. Having a high intake of antioxidants such as vitamin C, and especially vitamin E which is fat-soluble, protects cholesterol and other blood fats from damage.

Vitamin E is four times more effective at reducing the risk of a heart attack than the best available drug, according to Professor Morris Brown whose double-blind, controlled trial of vitamin E at Cambridge University Medical School showed a 75 per cent reduction in risk.[89] These results are consistent with those of two studies published in 1993. In one, which appeared in the *New England Journal of Medicine*, 87,200 nurses were given 100iu of vitamin E daily for more than two years. Forty per cent fewer heart attacks were reported amongst the subjects taking vitamin E, compared to those not taking vitamin E. In the other study 39,000 male health professionals were given 100iu of vitamin E for the same length of time; again there was a substantial 39 per cent reduction in heart attacks compared to those not taking vitamin E.[90] These results confirm the first reports of vitamin E's protective effect, made by Dr Evan Shute in the 1950s. Vitamin E also thins the blood, as do the omega-3 fish oils EPA and DHA which, in combination with vitamin E, are much more effective and considerably safer than aspirin.

Co-enzyme Q – the Missing Factor

Another nutrient, Co-enzyme Q, is showing miracle properties in helping patients with heart disease and other conditions in which energy production within cells is impaired. So astonishing are the properties of this nutrient that no fewer than 12 million people in Japan supplement their diets with Co-Q. In Kiev in the Ukraine a research institute has been set up solely to study the effects of this astonishing nutrient.

Co-Q was first isolated forty years ago in Britain by a group of scientists working in Liverpool, and was identified as a critical component in the production of energy within cells. The recent discovery that Co-Q is present in foods, that levels decline with age and that levels in cells rise when supplements are taken has led many scientists to consider Co-Q an undiscovered vitamin. Technically, Co-Q cannot be classified as a vitamin since it can be made by the body, even though it isn't made in large enough amounts for optimum health and energy. It is therefore a semi-essential nutrient.

Co-Q's magical properties lie in its ability to improve the cell's ability to use oxygen. In the most significant part of energy metabolism, when hydrogen reacts with oxygen, the latent energy in food is literally released as tiny charged particles called electrons. These are highly reactive and need to be very carefully handled. They are like nuclear fuel – a very potent, but very dangerous, energy source.

So dangerous are these spare electrons, also known as 'free radicals,' that, if not properly controlled, they are thought to be the initiating factor in making some cells cancerous and damaging artery walls, heralding heart disease. The damage caused to healthy cells by these spare electrons is a large part of what ageing is all about. The more damaged cells we have, the biochemically older we are. Compounds that contain spare electrons act as oxidants. They are created both during normal energy metabolism, and also by smoking, by eating fried food, by breathing in pollution, and through radiation from the sun.

Co-Q has two key roles to play in handling these volatile electrons. It controls the flow of oxygen, optimising the production of energy, and prevents damage caused by spare electrons. According to Dr Folkers, director of the Institute for Biomedical Research at Austin University in Texas, once body levels of Co-Q drop below 25 per cent of normal, disease may ensue.

In the last decade well over a hundred research trials have been conducted in the USA and Japan, with some astonishing results. Since Co-Q has such a critical part to play in the energy production of every single cell, its use in promoting health is far-reaching and perhaps best illustrated by recent trials on heart disease patients.

In a six-year study at the University of Texas involving people with congestive heart failure, a condition in which the heart, the largest muscle in the human body, becomes progressively weaker, 75 per cent of those on Co-Q survived three years, compared to 25 per cent on conventional medication.[91] In no fewer than twenty properly controlled studies published in the last two years Co-Q has repeatedly demonstrated a remarkable ability to improve heart function, and has now become the treatment of choice in Japan. In a combined trial by the University of Austin, Texas and the Centre for Adult Diseases in Osaka, Japan, 52 patients with high blood pressure were treated with either Co-Q or dummy tablets.[92] There was an 11 per cent decrease in blood pressure for those on Co-Q, compared to a 2 per cent decrease for those on dummy tablets.

Angina is a common condition in which sufferers experience pain in the heart region on exertion. It is usually caused by blockages in the tiny arteries that feed the heart muscle cells with oxygen. Since Co-Q helps all muscle cells to maximise their efficiency this magical nutrient has also been investigated as a natural treatment for angina. In one study at Hamamatsu University in Japan angina patients treated with Co-Q were able to take more exercise without feeling pain and had less frequent angina attacks.[93] After only four weeks on Co-Q other medication had effectively been halved.

Supernutrition for a Healthy Heart

Supplementing a combination of these nutrients is more effective in the long term than taking drugs designed to lower blood pressure; they deal with the cause of the problem, rather than the symptom. The chart below shows the levels to supplement, in addition to a good all-round multivitamin, both for basic prevention and for those at risk (with high blood pressure or a history of cardiovascular disease). It's also essential to change your diet by avoiding fried food and limiting your intake of meat and foods high in saturated fat, substituting carnivorous fish such as salmon, mackerel, herring and tuna. Eat plenty of fresh fruit, vegetables, nuts and seeds, which are high in calcium, magnesium and potassium. Avoid added salt, coffee and excess alcohol, don't smoke and keep yourself fit.

Supplement	For Basic Prevention	For Those at Risk
B6	10mg	50mg
Folic acid	400mcg	1000mcg
B12	10mcg	10mcg
Vitamin C	1000mg	2000–10000mg
Lysine	500mg	3000mg
Vitamin E	200ius	400–1000ius
EPA/DHA	300mg	1000mg
Co-enzyme Q10	30mg	90mg
Calcium	400mg	800mg
Magnesium	200mg	400mg

FOURTEEN

SAY NO TO INFLAMMATION

Many disease processes involve inflammation, which is often characterised by swelling, redness, pain and heat. These include all the 'itis' diseases such as arthritis, dermatitis, colitis, nephritis and hepatitis, as well as asthma and others not often associated with inflammation, for instance Alzheimer's and Parkinson's in which parts of the brain become inflamed. Inflammation also lies at the root of atherosclerosis, the common cause of thrombosis, heart attacks and strokes. It is an underlying cause of irritable bowel syndrome, Crohn's disease and ulcerative colitis, now suffered by 8 million people in Britain.

The most common medical treatment for inflammation is anti-inflammatory drugs. These fall into two categories: steroid hormones, usually derived from cortisone, such as Prednisone; and non-steroidal anti-inflammatory drugs, or NSAIDs for short, which include Ibuprofen, Voltarol, Naproxen and Diclofenac. These drugs are all effective painkillers but do nothing to address the causes of the inflammation. According to Dr Jeffrey Bland, a pioneer in new approaches to inflammation, 'instead of thinking "pain means drug", [we should think that] inflammation is the body's way of saying something is wrong. Inflammation is a "systemic" problem, not just a localised phenomenon, in which the body's physiology is shifted into an "alarm" state.' It's as if there is a series of underlying imbalances in the body's chemistry that build up and then burst forth once the body can no longer cope with a set of circumstances. The actual symptoms, or pain, is the wave breaking, although the wave is a long time coming.

From this perspective, there are several factors that set the scene for inflammation, and then those which trigger the manifestation of symptoms. So often it's the last straw that broke the camel's back that gets the blame: 'My eczema started when my marriage was breaking up', or 'ever since I had that bout of flu my joints have been aching.' These triggers are important and may include a trauma, an allergy, an infection, a toxin or exposure to too many oxidants. A healthy person can usually rise to such challenges; but if there are underlying weaknesses, such as a genetic predisposition or poor

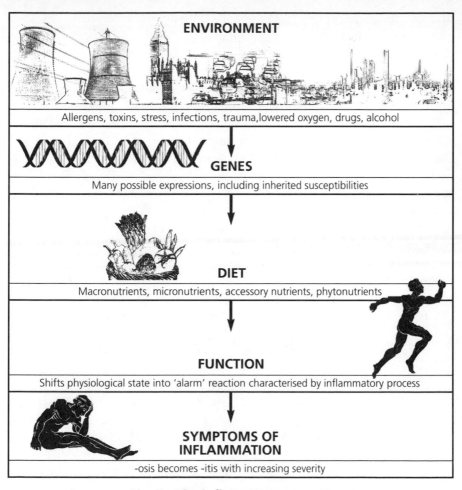

ENVIRONMENT

Allergens, toxins, stress, infections, trauma,lowered oxygen, drugs, alcohol

GENES

Many possible expressions, including inherited susceptibilities

DIET

Macronutrients, micronutrients, accessory nutrients, phytonutrients

FUNCTION

Shifts physiological state into 'alarm' reaction characterised by inflammatory process

SYMPTOMS OF INFLAMMATION

-osis becomes -itis with increasing severity

Fig. 8   The inflammatory process

nutritional status, that person may have no reserves in his or her health bank and so even the slightest stress cannot be accommodated. All these factors need to be considered when attempting to restore health.

Toxic Overload

Inflammation is the body's way of showing that a person's intake from the environment, including diet, drugs and environmental chemicals, has exceeded their capacity to adapt. Take asthma, for example: the incidence has gone up dramatically among children; the annual death rate among twenty-four-year-olds more than doubled between 1980 and 1993; the percentage that have to receive hospital treatment has gone up by 28 per cent. This is, in part, related to increased exposure to air pollutants such as ozone, sulphur dioxide, acid aerosols and indoor cigarette smoke as well as other toxins in pesticide residues, medication, food and water. In the excellent book *Our Stolen Future*, Dr Theo Colborn and colleagues investigated the impact on human reproduction of the cocktail of eighty thousand chemicals to which we are typically exposed in the West. They found that toxic chemicals can mimic or block hormones which get inside the nucleus of the cell and literally change genetic expression – they reprogram you. Dr Arnold and colleagues reported in the journal *Science*[94] their study of two such xeno–oestrogens (oestrogen mimickers). Combined, they were a thousand times more disrupting than in isolation. What, you may wonder, is the combined effect of the thousands of chemicals we are all unwittingly exposed to? Nobody knows.

The key factors that contribute to developing an inflammatory health problem are:

- Impaired liver detoxification
- Disturbed blood sugar control
- Too many oxidants and not enough antioxidants
- Lack of essential fats
- Allergy

How Strong Is Your Liver?

As a gastroenterologist from Harvard Medical School said, 'A good stomach and set of bowels is more important to human health and happiness than a large amount of brains.' The scene for inflammation may be set in the digestive tract where faulty nutrition can result in dysbiosis, a disruption of healthy gut bacteria, leading to bacterial, fungal or parasite infection, intestinal permeability and allergy. Once the gut wall becomes leaky more proteins than normal get into the bloodstream, initiating allergic reactions. Along with other toxins, they tax the liver's ability to detoxify. Once the liver's reserve is impaired, any dietary or environmental insult can trigger inflammation. This whole process of digestive problems leading to liver overload is a common cause of chronic fatigue syndrome and is explained more fully in Chapter 17.

The good news is that each of these factors can be tested by a nutrition consultant and corrected. Specific nutrients help to improve liver function. These include antioxidants, certain amino acids and phytochemicals found in natural, unadulterated foods. Brussels sprouts are a case in point. Naturally rich in the phytochemicals known as glucosinolates, Brussels sprouts gained their reputation as an anti-cancer food. Three servings a day have been reported to halve the risk of some cancers.[95] In a double-blind controlled trial one group of participants were given normal sprouts to eat, while the other group had sprouts with the glucosinolates removed. Eating 300g of the normal sprouts a day increased the activity of an important liver enzyme, glutathione S-transferase (GST), by as much as 30 per cent.

Anyone with a long-term inflammatory problem, from arthritis to asthma, is likely to benefit by seeing a nutrition consultant, having a liver detoxification test, and adjusting their diet and supplements accordingly. This alone can make a real difference.

Are You Insulin-dependent?

There is a strong link between many of the signs of inflammation and being resistant to insulin, the hormone produced by the pancreas that helps to control blood sugar levels. Most diabetics are 'insulin-resistant' in that their body doesn't react to insulin in the way that it should. Insulin is released into the bloodstream whenever you eat carbohydrates, especially sugar, or stimulants. The insulin then helps to transport the glucose from carbohydrates into body cells. But this doesn't happen if you are insulin-resistant, a biochemical characteristic not limited to diabetics. Linked with insulin resistance, sometimes called Syndrome X, is an increased risk for diabetes, polycystic ovaries, hypertension (high blood pressure), high levels of cholesterol and triglycerides, obesity, breast cancer, stroke, cardiovascular disease and sugar cravings. (See Chapter 17 for a full discussion of this syndrome.)

As a consequence of Syndrome X, glucose levels in the blood stay too high and cells become 'sugar-coated'. Too much glucose or insulin in the blood is toxic and triggers inflammatory reactions. In the cells, a disturbed glucose supply acts as a powerful oxidant, damaging cells, as well as producing the symptom of fatigue and triggering, amongst other reactions, inflammation. Amyloid proteins, associated with both insulin resistance and inflammation, are found in the blockages in blood vessels that trigger a heart attack. This has led to the realisation that atherosclerosis is also, in part, an inflammatory disease.

Insulin resistance can be tested (see Chapter 17). Once it has been identified, the major way of restoring balance is through diet and supplements. From a dietary point of view, the following three factors are most important:

- eat more fibre in wholefoods, particularly soluble fibres such as those found in oats, beans and vegetables

- eat foods which release their sugar content slowly: that means wholegrains, oats, lentils, beans, apples and raw or lightly cooked vegetables

- take the following daily supplements: vitamin C (1000mg), vitamin E (400mg), magnesium (400mg), chromium (200mcg) and essential fats, especially the fish oil EPA.

Oxidants vs Antioxidants

Any inflammation indicates a state of alarm in the body. One of the primary defence weapons is oxidants, but these can also harm the body and initiate inflammation. It's a vicious loop. Oxidants are produced by the body in the mitochondria, the cell's energy factories, which turn glucose from food into energy. These oxidants, which are much like toxic exhaust from an engine, must be rendered harmless by antioxidants such as vitamins A, C and E. Too many oxidants and not enough antioxidants can lead to cell damage. The liver, too, produces oxidants if its detoxifying capacity has been exceeded.

Another self-made oxidant is nitric oxide. While it plays some important roles in the body, levels can become excessive if the immune system is on red alert, perhaps due to frequent consumption of an allergen or breathing in toxins. Body levels tend to be higher at times of inflammation, and high levels of nitric oxide have been linked to arthritis, asthma and migraine.

We also put oxidants into our bodies by eating fried food, or by breathing smoke-filled or polluted air. These can damage the gut and/or the lungs, leading to greater susceptibility to infection as well as inflammation.

The goal is therefore to calm down the immune system, avoid allergens, take away sources of oxidants and add antioxidant nutrients. In addition to the traditional antioxidants vitamins A, C and E, selenium and zinc, two other substances can help reduce inflammation: the mineral magnesium and quercitin, which is derived from dimorphandra, a type of rhododendron. The latter two are particularly helpful for dealing with asthma.

In chronic inflammatory conditions, the energy factories of cells can become extensively damaged, leading to chronic fatigue and to aches and pains as experienced in fibromyalgia or rheumatoid arthritis. These impaired mitochondria can, however, be brought back to life by supplying the body with the kind of nutrients that help rebuild them. These include the amino acids reduced glutathione, n-acetyl cysteine and n-acetyl carnitine, plus vitamin E, lipoic acid and co-enzyme Q. Niacinamide may also be helpful and has certainly proved so for arthritis sufferers, according to the work of Dr Kaufman. He successfully treated thousands of patients with it in the 1960s – a practice which proved to help arthritics in a recent double-blind controlled trial.[96] Glucosamine is another valuable nutrient for those with arthritis, while the amino acid glutamine is especially important in inflammatory conditions of the gut, such as Crohn's disease, irritable bowel syndrome and colitis, and in similar conditions of the brain, including

Alzheimer's. As well as healing the gut, glutamine also helps to rebuild joints and to improve memory. All these supplements are available in health food stores, although it is wiser to work with a nutritionist who can assess exactly what you need, devise a suitable supplement programme and save you spending more than you need.

Nature's Anti-inflammatories

Frankincense may be the ultimate gift for an arthritic friend. More precisely, *Boswellia serrata*, also known as Indian frankincense, which is proving to be a very powerful natural anti-inflammatory agent without the side-effects of current drugs. Anti-inflammatory and painkilling drugs such as aspirin and phenylbutazone irritate the digestive tract, causing symptoms in over 20 per cent of long-term users. They work by blocking the body's ability to produce inflammatory chemicals from dietary fats. But boswellic acids contained within the herb achieve comparable anti-inflammatory effects without the associated gut problems. Trials with arthritic patients have shown significant relief after four weeks of supplementing a daily 600mg of boswellic acid.[97] Preparations are available in tablet and cream form in the USA and are becoming available in the UK. The creams are expecially useful in the treatment of localised inflammation, such as arthritis.

Another natural anti-inflammatory agent occurs in turmeric and mustard, both rich sources of substances called curcumins. Extracts of turmeric have been found to have powerful antioxidant and anti-inflammatory properties. Trials on arthritic patients have again shown improvement of a similar order to that offered by the anti-inflammatory drugs, and again without the side-effects.[98] Curcumins have a similar mode of action to boswellic acid and, together with a good optimum nutrition programme including anti-inflammatory essential fats, may prove at least as effective as drugs.

Anti-inflammatory Fats

The essential fats from seeds and fish have proved most helpful in a wide variety of inflammatory conditions from asthma to arthritis. Most effective are sources of gamma-linolenic acid (GLA), which is a member of the omega-6 family of essential fats. GLA is naturally rich in evening primrose oil and borage (starflower) oil. Supplementing 300mg of GLA daily (equivalent to 3000mg of evening primrose oil) has been shown to be as effective in the treatment of arthritis as anti-inflammatory drugs.[99]

The value of fish oils high in the omega-3 family of fats, particularly EPA and DHA, is well established in fighting inflammation. Like GLA, these essential fats are the building blocks for the body's natural anti-inflammatory agents, known as prostaglandins. Without them the body's chemistry tilts towards inflammation. Numerous studies have reported less swelling, pain and tenderness after supplementing concentrated fish oils containing 1–3g EPA.[100] These natural anti-inflammatory fats are particularly rich in fish with teeth, which eat fish that eat plankton. Each step up the food chain concentrates the fats. To experience their benefit, either supplement 1–3g EPA daily or eat salmon, mackerel, herring or tuna three times a week.

However, a word of caution: if you have a very poor intake of antioxidant nutrients and are generating a lot of oxidants due to inflammation, these essential fats can be oxidised and may worsen the condition. Under these conditions it is best to restore the oxidant–antioxidant balance by first eliminating allergens and adding antioxidant nutrients for a month. Only then should you add in anti-inflammatory fish oils (omega-3 fats) and evening primrose or borage oil (omega-6 fats).

Eliminating Allergies

Most people with inflammatory diseases have allergies to certain foods or chemicals. These allergies may occur because of an inflamed gut wall, which becomes permeable to large food proteins. Once these get into the body they trigger an allergic response, which includes inflammation. The most common intestinal irritants are dairy produce, wheat and other grains, eggs, beef, chilli, coffee and peanuts. One way to reduce the load on the digestive system and to test for allergies is to avoid these foods for twenty days. An excellent 'self-help' diet is explained in *The 20 Day Rejuvenation Diet Program* by Dr Jeffrey Bland.

At the end of the twenty days reintroduce these foods one by one, noting any symptoms that occur within twenty-four hours of eating that food. This may indicate which foods, if any, you are intolerant to. A more thorough approach is to have what is known as a Quantitative ELISA IgG allergy test, which involves giving a blood sample from which your sensitivity to a hundred foods is tested (see Useful Addresses). Supplementing key gut-restoring nutrients while avoiding allergy-provoking foods will help to heal the gut, reduce allergic potential, lessen the load on the liver and immune system and reduce inflammation.

Restoring the Balance

This new approach to conquering inflammation is best tackled by working with a qualified nutrition consultant who can run the necessary tests and advise you on diet and supplements for each stage of reprograming your body. It is, as already explained, based on an understanding that inflammation and pain are the body's way of saying 'Help!' and that current diet and lifestyle factors have exceeded the body's capacity to adapt. Restoring the balance can normally be achieved in three to six months and involves:

Reducing environmental toxins including drugs, alcohol and environmental pollutants

Testing your liver detoxification potential by seeing a nutrition consultant who can devise a nutritional strategy to improve your ability to detoxify (see Chapter 17)

Balancing your blood sugar   Avoid all sugar and stimulants and reduce stress. Eat slow-releasing carbohydrates and high-fibre foods. Supplement vitamins C and E, magnesium and chromium

Reducing oxidants and increasing antioxidants   Avoid smoking and fried foods and supplement a comprehensive antioxidant formula

Supplementing natural anti-inflammatory agents including glucosamine, quercitin, boswellic acid or curcumin.

Increasing your intake of essential fats by eating cold-pressed seed oils and fish or supplementing GLA (from evening primrose or borage oil) and EPA/DHA (from fish oils)

Identifying and avoiding allergens either by having an IgG ELISA Allergy test or by avoiding highly allergenic foods for twenty days.

FIFTEEN

DEVELOPING SUPER-IMMUNITY

The greatest threat to face mankind in the twenty-first century may not be nuclear war, pollution, starvation or infertility, but the danger from infections. The signs are there already – a doubling of death rates from infectious diseases in the 1990s; new viruses with no apparent cure; new strains of bacteria resistant to antibiotics. Is nature beating us at our own game? Will medical science keep developing new drugs to treat immune disease? Or are we missing the point?

We owe much to Louis Pasteur, whose research established that micro-organisms were a source of infection. He fought hard to get this message across, and it wasn't until after his death that the full impact of his work became clear. At the time he said, 'If anyone should say that my conclusions go beyond established facts, I would agree, in the sense that I have taken a stand unreservedly on an order of ideas which, strictly speaking, cannot be irrefutably demonstrated.' Here we stand, more than a century later, in much the same position, with an order of ideas that points clearly to a new direction in medicine and healthcare.

Even before his death, Pasteur had shifted his focus on disease from the invader to the host. Perhaps we are not the innocent victim. Perhaps our susceptibility has as much to do with the health of our own immune system as it does to exposure to viruses, bacteria or parasites. Instead of focussing solely on killing the invader, perhaps we should be looking at how to strengthen our own defences.

To C or Not to C?

That's the thinking that drew Linus Pauling into immunology, a field much transformed by his insights. By 1965 he had become fascinated with vitamin C. Here was a substance that at 10mg a day prevented scurvy and at 10,000mg a day held back cancer with no toxicity even at levels ten times higher. Vitamin C, he discovered, was produced by almost all animals at levels at least fifteen times greater than daily human consumption. What's more, vitamin C-producing animals were immune to many viral diseases, including pulmonary tuberculosis, diptheria, a viral form of leukaemia and poliomyelitis.[101] Could it be, he pondered, that mankind's susceptibility to infections was in part due to a shortage of vitamin C?

In 1965 he and his wife started taking 3g of vitamin C daily to see whether it would prevent everyday infections, including colds.

> We realised that it did apparently protect us from the common cold. I no longer had these miserable colds that used to plague me every few months during my whole previous life. I decided to write a book *Vitamin C and the Common Cold* which was published in 1970. It was a best-seller and received the Phi Beta Kappa Award for best scientific book of the year.
>
> I checked the medical literature to find out what evidence there was at that time. I found four well-conducted controlled trials involving what I would describe now as rather small amounts of vitamin C. The best was a randomised double-blind trial by Dr Ritzel, the physician for a school system in Basle, Switzerland. He gave boys at a winter camp either half a gram of vitamin C or a placebo. There was 63 per cent less illness with the common cold in those taking vitamin C.

Many years later Professor Hemila, a Professor of Medicine in Helsinki, Finland, came across Pauling's book and decided to check the medical literature to find out how many studies had been carried out since 1970.[17] He decided that he would only accept randomised, double-blind studies in which at least 1g was given, and found thirty-eight clinical trials that satisfied these requirements. 'Randomised' means people are randomly put into either the group taking vitamin C or the group taking a placebo. 'Double-blind' means, for the duration of the test, neither the participants nor the experimenters know who is taking what, so there is no risk of bias. Thirty-seven of the 38 studies concluded that vitamin C has a protective effect greater than placebo, and a dozen had high statistical significance, at $p=0.001$. That means there is 99.9 per cent confidence that the results weren't due to chance.

As far as Pauling, who died in 1994 at the age of ninety-three, was concerned. 'There is no doubt that vitamin C in large doses has value against the common cold. My recommendation is not 1 gram a day, but to take 1 or 2 grams every hour at the first sign of a cold as long as symptoms still persist. Keep doing that until you forget because the symptoms have gone away. This will stop a cold in almost everyone who follows the regimen.'

Since then, vitamin C has been proved effective against a broad range of viruses, including HIV. It also has many other immune-boosting roles. It stimulates formation of T-lymphocytes, which are important immune cells, and calms down inflammation by enhancing prostaglandin formation from essential fats. It is also antibacterial and a natural antihistamine, as well as helping to neutralise bacterial toxins. It improves the performance of anti-bodies involved in allergic responses and stimulates non-lysosyme antibacterial factor (NLAF), mononuclear phagocytes and leucocytes – other key components of the immune system.

Immune Connections

Yet vitamin C is but one of many known ways to build up your defences. Other important immune boosters include vitamin A and betacarotene, B6, zinc, selenium and the amino acids glutathione and cysteine.

Immune Boosting Nutrients

Vitamin A is especially important because it helps to maintain the integrity of the digestive tract, lungs and all cell membranes, preventing foreign substances from entering the body, or viruses from entering cells. In addition, vitamin A and betacarotene are potent antioxidants; many foreign substances produce free oxidising radicals (oxidants) as part of their defence system. Macrophages, a type of immune cell, also produce free radicals to destroy invaders. A high intake of antioxidant nutrients helps to protect immune cells from these harmful weapons. The ideal daily intake of betacarotene is between 10,000ius (3300mcgRE) and 30,000ius (10,000mcgRE).

Vitamins B5, B6, B12 and folic acid are all important to the immune system. The production of antibodies and the function of T-lymphocytes depends on B6, so it's essential when fighting an infection. The ideal daily intake is 50–100mg. B12 and folic acid are important for the same reasons, the ideal daily intake being 100mcg for B12 and 400mcg for folic acid. Pantothenic acid (B5) deficiency is associated with inhibition of T-cell and antibody production. The ideal daily intake is 100–300mg.

Vitamin C is unquestionably the master immune-boosting nutrient with more than a dozen proven immune-boosting roles. During a viral infection saturation with vitamin C prevents viruses from multiplying. 'Saturation' usually involves daily doses of 10g or more, spread throughout the day. That's more than a hundred times the Recommended Daily Allowance (RDA) – the level set by the government to prevent scurvy! Fortunately, as already explained, vitamin C is one of the least toxic substances known to man.

Vitamin E is another important all-rounder, vitamin E improves B- and T-cell function and is a powerful antioxidant. Its immune-boosting properties increase when given in conjunction with selenium. The ideal daily intake is 400–800ius.

Selenium, zinc, manganese, copper and zinc are all involved in antioxidation and all have been shown to affect immune power positively. Of these, selenium and zinc are the most important. Zinc is critical for immune cell production and function of B- and T-cells. Selenium boosts immunity and works synergistically with vitamin E. Ideal daily doses are 100–200mcg. The ideal daily intake of zinc is 15–50mg (short-term only). While zinc supplementation above 15mg a day may be beneficial during a viral infection, it's not such a good idea during a bacterial infection because bacteria do better on zinc too. The same is true for iron: while iron deficiency suppresses immune function, too much interferes with the ability of macrophages to destroy bacteria. When an infection is present, the body initiates a series of defence mechanisms designed to stop the invader absorbing iron, so during a bacterial infection iron supplementation may actually hinder the immune system.

One of the big breakthroughs in recent years has been the way in which viral diseases may develop as a consequence of sub-optimum nutrition, and then pave the way for further diseases to develop. The presence of herpes infection, for example, has been identified as a risk factor for developing Alzheimer's later in life.[102] Recent research by Dr Orville Levander from the US government's Nutrients Requirements and Functions Laboratory found that, when an animal is low in both vitamin E and selenium and exposed to a virus, the virus is able to change form more readily and become more harmful.[103] Viruses also interfere with our own immune defences by preventing immune cells from becoming specialised members of the immune army, a measure which vitamin C counteracts.

Keeping the body topped up with enough vitamin C, E and selenium not only makes it difficult for a virus to survive, but renders it much less harmful. This synergism between nutrients may prove to be the way forward for deep-rooted infections.

HIV – think positive

AIDS is a case in point. It is considered by many to be the inevitable and usually fatal consequence of HIV infection. Over the last few years a growing body of evidence has shown that HIV-infected people and AIDS patients exhibit nutritional deficiencies which may contribute to the underlying immune suppression. Doctors have consistently reported improvement when patients were given nutrient supplements.

Nutritional supplementation therefore is likely to play a significant role in the management of HIV and AIDS, according to Dr Raxit Jariwalla, head of Immunodeficiency Research at the Linus Pauling Institute of Science and Medicine.[104] His research has shown that vitamin C is more effective in suppressing HIV in infected human cells than the drug AZT. He showed that both vitamin C and AZT can block the new infection of cells, but AZT, unlike vitamin C, has no effect on virus production in cells which are already chronically infected. Vitamin C alone was 99 per cent effective in inactivating the virus. Around 10g of vitamin C a day halved virus activity, while twice as much antiviral protection was achieved by combining vitamin C with the amino acid N-acetyl-cysteine.

N-acetyl-cysteine, which can be converted by the body into glutathione, is a very potent immune stimulator, especially in people with deep-rooted infections in which there is substantial cell damage. The combination of high-dose vitamin C (10–40g a day) with 3–5g N-acetyl-cysteine may prove to be the backbone of future treatment for those who are HIV-postive. At the time of writing Dr Jariwalla, in conjunction with the US National Institutes of Health, is due to test this approach by giving vitamin C and N-acetyl-cysteine to people who are HIV-positive and recording the outcome. I have certainly found that these nutrients, plus other important immune boosters, can restore immune T-cell counts to normal HIV-positive people who exhibit no AIDS symptoms.

It is interesting to note that the leading edge of drug treatment for AIDS involves the combination of many drugs that both give the HIV virus a hard time and prevent the opportunistic infections that develop. In the same light, I believe we will find that the combined use of nutrients will prove equally, if not more powerful, without the risk of side-effects.

Synergistic Vitamins

The power of combining immune-boosting nutrients was demonstrated by an experiment by leading immunologist Ranjit Chandra of the Memorial Univesity of Newfoundland.[15] He gave 96 healthy, elderly men and women either a multivitamin and mineral supplement or a dummy pill. After a year, those taking the supplement had halved their incidence of infections. Chandra also found objective proof that the supplement had boosted their immune power: when he measured immune activity, he found that T-lymphocytes, natural killer cells and antibodies were all responding more efficiently.

Helpful Herbs

Aloe vera is a powerful detoxifier and antiseptic with immune-boosting and antiviral properties. Exactly what the 'active ingredient' is remains a bit of a mystery. Aloe vera is rich in mucopolysaccharides, one of which is called acemannan, and also contains lignins, enzymes, antiseptic agents, vitamins, minerals and amino acids.

Cat's claw is a powerful antiviral, antioxidant and immune-boosting agent from the Peruvian rainforest plant *Uncaria tomentosa*. It contains alkaloids including isopteridin, which has been proven to boost immune function. Cat's claw is available as a tea or in supplements. As a tea it tastes good with added blackcurrant and apple concentrate. To fight an infection you need 2–4g a day, or four cups of tea. One cup of cat's claw tea a day helps maintain immune power.

Echinacea is another great all-rounder with antiviral and antibacterial properties. It's the original Native American snakeroot which later became known as snake oil. The active ingredients are thought to be specific mucopolysaccharides. It comes in capsules and in extracts, taken as drops. To fight an infection you need 2–3g a day, or 15 drops three times a day, of concentrated echinacea extract.

Elderberry extract, also known as Sambucol, is an antiviral agent: it prevents viruses from penetrating cells, which they need to do in order to replicate themselves. A dessertspoon three times a day has been shown to effect complete relief from certain strains of influenza in 73 per cent of patients within two days and 90 per cent within three days.[105]

Garlic contains allicin, which is antiviral, antifungal and antibacterial. It also acts as an antioxidant, being rich in sulphur-containing amino acids. To fight an infection you need 2–4 cloves a day or the equivalent in capsules.

Grapefruit seed extract, also called Citricidal, is a powerful antiviral, antifungal and antibiotic agent but does not have anything like the damaging effect on the beneficial gut bacteria as conventional antibiotics do. Even so, if you're taking probiotics (such as *acidophilus*) it's best to take them separately from the grapefruit seed extract. It comes in drop form and can be swallowed, gargled or used as nose drops or ear drops, depending on the site of infection. To fight an infection you need 10 drops, two or three times a day.

Immune-boosting Herbs

The three most potent immune-boosting herbs are echinacea, cat's claw and garlic. Garlic is worth including in your daily diet. It contains significant levels of cysteine, an important antioxidant which also has broad antiviral, antibacterial and antifungal properties. Eat a clove a day – more if you're fighting an infection – or consider a garlic supplement. Aloe vera is another good all-round tonic which stimulates the production of immune cells and improves their function, among other benefits.

Echinacea and cat's claw are best reserved for fighting infections, or for short-term immune system boosts – for example, when on holiday. Both contain alkaloids, which boost the immune system and stimulate phagocytosis (the ability of white blood cells to attack and digest invaders), as well as cancer cells. A word of warning, however. The effects of these alkaloids, especially in large amounts, has not been properly tested in pregnancy.

How to Boost Your Immune System

The best way to keep your immune system strong and able to adapt in an unhealthy environment is to:

- eat a diet rich in fruit, vegetables, nuts, seeds and wholefoods

- stay away from fried foods, foods high in saturated fat (that means less meat and dairy produce and more fish), alcohol, coffee and cigarettes, all of which are potent immune suppressors

- avoid prolonged stress or a lack of sleep, which also weaken your immune system

In addition, supplement the following on a daily basis:

- a good all-round multivitamin and mineral (check what your multi provides and top up accordingly with additional supplements)
- vitamin C – 2000mg
- vitamin A – 7500ius (2500mcgRE)
- betacarotene – 15,000iu (5000mcgRE)
- vitamin E – 400ius
- selenium – 100mcg
- zinc – 20mg
- manganese – 5mg
- daily garlic
- optional aloe vera

When fighting an infection double all these doses (NB during pregnancy vitamin A should not exceed 10,000ius/3000mcg) and start taking 2 grams of vitamin C every four hours. Also take cat's claw tea or capsules plus 10 drops of echinacea extract three times a day.

If you have a cold or flu add to the above medications a dessertspoon of Sambucol (elderberry extract), three times a day. For stomach bugs, bladder infections, and bacterial and fungal infections take 10 drops Citricidal (grapefruit seed extract) three times a day; gargle with it if you have a sore throat.

SIXTEEN

SOLVING SUGAR SENSITIVITY

Nothing is more critical for human health than sugar. Sugar, or more precisely glucose, is the fuel from which we make energy. Consequently, the ability to control the balance of glucose in the body and to release its energy potential determines our physical and mental energy levels. The brain, which consumes about a quarter of the energy we derive from food, needs the most glucose, followed by the liver and the skeletal muscles. The rest is used by the heart, the immune system and other organs.

Conventional medicine used to recognise only one type of sugar imbalance – diabetes. Now we know that there are subtle stages of sugar imbalance which may prove a major predictor of health problems and that diabetes may be simply the last stage.

Two Kinds of Diabetes

Diabetes is a condition in which blood sugar levels are high as a result of the body's inability to transport excess sugar from the blood into body cells for storage. For glucose (the end product of carbohydrate digestion), the blood is merely a mode of transport into the cells, so excess blood glucose means there's not enough in the cells; this results in mental and physical exhaustion and black-outs.

There are two main kinds of diabetes, with distinctly different causes, now suffered by 1.4 million people in the UK. The first, called child-onset diabetes or insulin-dependent diabetes (IDD), tends to strike in the early teenage years, although the incidence is increasing in children under five years old. In the UK there are around twenty thousand people under the age of twenty who inject themselves with insulin. It starts with the immune system destroying the pancreatic cells that produce insulin, but exactly why this occurs has long been a mystery.

The second type, adult diabetes, also known as diabetes mellitus or non-insulin-dependent diabetes is primarily caused by, and treated through diet.

The main culprit is sugar. A third, transient, kind of diabetes can also occur during pregnancy.

Child Diabetes Linked to Milk Allergy

While there is a genetic predisposition to insulin-dependent diabetes, this is only part of the picture. Another factor is suggested by findings that genetically susceptible children who had been partly breastfed for at least seven months or exclusively breastfed for at least three or four months had a significantly decreased incidence of IDD. Children who have not been exposed to cow's milk until four months or older also show the same substantially reduced risk. The highest incidence of IDD is found in Finland, which has the world's highest milk product consumption.

Animal studies showed that rats bred to be susceptible to diabetes had a much higher risk if their feed contained either milk or wheat gluten. In one study even the addition of 1 per cent skimmed milk increased the incidence of IDD from 15 per cent to 52 per cent. In 1993 Dr Hans-Michael Dosch, Professor of Immunology at Mount Sinai Hospital, New York, identified the specific factor in dairy produce, known as bovine serum albumin (BSA), that increased the risk of diabetes; he showed that it cross-reacted with pancreatic cells. Dosch theorised that, if children susceptible to diabetes are introduced to BSA before they are four months old (when the gut wall is immature and more permeable), they would develop an allergic response to BSA in which immune cells would mistakenly destroy not only the BSA molecules but also pancreatic tissue. He went on to show that, of 142 newly diagnosed IDD children, 100 per cent of them had antibodies to BSA – in other words they were allergic to it – compared to 2 per cent of non-diabetic children. Dr Dosch believes that the presence of these anti-BSA antibodies can predict child-onset diabetes in 80–90 per cent of cases.

With this evidence, he believes that keeping all babies off dairy products for at least their first six months halves the risk of IDD. BSA can, however, pass from the mother's diet into breast milk. So if breastfeeding mothers avoid beef and dairy products this may remove the risk completely in genetically susceptible children. The current opinion is that about 1 in 4 children are genetically susceptible but only at risk of developing diabetes if certain dietary or environmental triggers are present. While early introduction to dairy food, leading to a BSA allergy, is one such trigger, it is unlikely to be the only factor.

Adult Diabetes is 90 Per Cent Diet

The average sugar intake in Britain has risen from the equivalent of two teaspoons a day in the 1820s to thirty-eight teaspoons a day in the 1980s. Such major changes in diet place a significant stress on the body's ability to adapt. In fact it's a wonder that only 10 per cent of the population develop diabetes when you take into account not only this rise in sugar consumption but also the general decrease in dietary fibre, which helps to slow down the release of food's natural sugar into the bloodstream, and the widespread deficiency of the numerous vitamins and minerals that are needed to digest, transport and make use of sugar. The complications of diabetes are blindness, kidney disease, cardiovascular disease and nerve damage. The third most common cause of death in the West is from these complications, particularly cardio-vascular disease.

Are you dysglycemic?

New evidence is supporting the view that adult diabetes is a long time coming. Before diabetes ever develops, a person may have varying levels of dysglycemia – imbalances in blood sugar control. This starts manifesting as insulin resistance – an insensitivity to the hormone. When we eat carbo-hydrate foods the body produces insulin to help carry the glucose out of the bloodstream. Yet according to Dr Gerald Reaven, Professor of Medicine at Stanford University, California, who pioneered research in the 1980s, 'Insulin resistance is present in the majority of patients with impaired glu-cose tolerance or non-insulin-dependent diabetes and in approximately 25 per cent of non-obese individuals with normal oral glucose tolerance.'[106] That means that you have at least a 25 per cent chance of being insulin-resistant and, as a result, a reduced ability to keep your blood sugar level even. Symptoms include weakness, fatigue, dizziness, nervousness, irritabil-ity and difficulty in concentrating. This syndrome is also linked to obesity

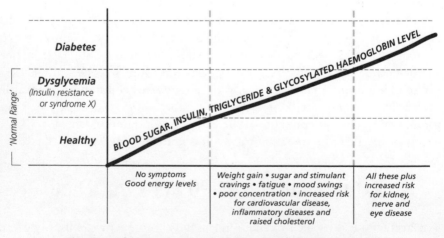

Fig. 9   Where are you on the scale of sugar control?

and cravings for sugar or stimulants such as sweet foods, chocolate, coffee, tea or cigarettes. Obesity develops because the body's metabolism is unable to get glucose out of the blood effectively and learns how to store it as fat. A person with such an altered metabolism only needs to look at food to gain weight. Ironically, such people, packed full of energy in the form of fat, get none of the benefit and often feel tired all the time.

Insulin resistance, also known as Syndrome X, has far-reaching health implications as it is associated with cardiovascular disease, raised cholesterol, inflammatory diseases, gout and, eventually, adult diabetes. That's the bad news. The good news is that by optimising your blood sugar control you also reduce your risk of all of these major causes of premature death in the Western world.

Testing for Syndrome X

While conventional checks for diabetes (which involve measuring your blood sugar level after an intake of sugar, for example a sweetened drink) will determine if you have diabetes, they don't pick up Syndrome X and therefore aren't an effective early warning signal. However, simultaneously measuring insulin levels in the blood can diagnose the syndrome. If insulin is high and glucose is marginally high two hours after consuming a measured amount of glucose, this indicates insulin resistance. It shows that the insulin isn't working properly, which is why the blood sugar levels stay high and why the body keeps producing insulin. Another blood test, which is more accurate, involves 'glycosylated' haemoglobin – it measures the extent to which your red blood cells have become sugar-coated. If your blood sugar level is frequently too high because your cells are resistant to insulin then the red blood cells start to get coated in glucose. Both these tests are available from your GP.

Sugar – the greatest toxin

Despite being the most important nutrient of all, sugar is highly toxic. It is an oxidant – in other words it oxidises or damages certain substances, especially proteins. The toxic by-product of glucose is known as AGE (advanced glycosylation end products) and, ironically, that's exactly what they do. If there's too much glucose floating around it damages cells and makes them age faster. AGE also damages blood fats, impairing the ability of the body to remove unwanted cholesterol, and collagen, making the skin less elastic.

While most cells require the presence of fully-functioning insulin to take in glucose, there are three that don't – the kidneys, eyes and nerves. In both Syndrome X and diabetes they become overloaded with glucose, which is why the complications of the disease so often include blindness, kidney disease and nerve damage. The risk of these complications can be more than halved by controlling the glucose levels in diabetics.[107]

The dangers of too much insulin

Insulin is a very powerful body chemical and you don't want too much in the bloodstream: it encourages the formation of stress hormones from the adrenal glands while depressing the formation of DHEA, a hormone that helps to protect from stress. So the end result of too much insulin is lowered ability to tolerate stress. Excessive insulin also stimulates the formation of testosterone, which disturbs the balance of the sex hormones and can increase upper body and abdominal fat.

Glucose tolerance factor

Insulin doesn't, however, work alone. It is both made and helped by an adequate supply of key vitamins and minerals. Vitamin B6 and the mineral zinc are needed for its formation, while the presence of chromium greatly increases its efficiency. Chromium deficiency therefore forces the body to work harder to produce more insulin. Adult diabetics have lower chromium levels than non-diabetics[108] and, if given chromium, show improved glucose tolerance.[109] The average diet provides only about 30mcg of chromium a day; large amounts are lost when food is refined – 90 per cent of it goes from flour, rice or sugar. So only a wholefood diet is likely to provide enough of this essential element, with ideal intakes estimated at 50–200mcg a day. What's more, people with insulin resistance, perhaps due to too much sugar, stimulants or stress, use up chromium at a much faster rate and so become deficient.

Deficiency also increases with age. Research by Dr Stephen Davies and colleagues at the Biolab Medical Unit in London analysed 51,665 samples of hair, blood and sweat taken from 40,872 patients and found a clear, age-related decline in chromium levels: seventy-five-year-olds had almost half the levels of chromium as children aged one to four.[110] This pattern of ever-decreasing levels is strongly suggestive of a nationwide diet that fails to meet adequate levels.

Supplementing 200mcg of chromium a day can really help even out blood sugar levels, decrease insulin requirement, lower blood cholesterol and triglycerides and increase the cholesterol remover HDL.[111]

Solving sugar sensitivity

Knowing where you are along the path from normal glucose control to insulin resistance, and finally to diabetes, is one of the best ways to test for and promote functional health. Since the primary causes of problems here are dietary, changing what you eat is the place to start for both prevention and control of blood sugar imbalance. And since improved sugar control is consistent with an improved ability to maintain high energy levels, these recommendations are an essential part of an action plan for high energy living.

- Avoid or substantially reduce all use of stimulants and depressants including coffee, tea, chocolate, cigarettes and alcohol. This is particularly important for those who show signs of an addictive pattern of consumption, i.e. having regular intakes of tea or coffee every day.

- Eat wholefoods as much as possible. That means brown rice, brown bread, wholewheat pasta and naturally whole foods such as nuts, seeds, lentils, beans, vegetables and fruit.

- Make sure most of the carbohydrate foods you eat are 'low glycemic index' foods – ones that release their glucose content slowly, such as apples, oats, wholegrains, lentils, beans, tofu and raw vegetables.

- For people with symptoms of dysglycemia, blood sugar levels can be kept more constant by eating low-fat protein alongside carbohydrates. This means, for example, having some nuts with a piece of fruit, or tofu or fish with rice or pasta.

- Supplement vitamins C and B complex, which are needed for proper energy metabolism (a high dose B complex plus 2000mg of vitamin C a day).

- Supplement antioxidants (an all-round antioxidant formula) to prevent cell damage through the formation of the toxic by-products of glucose.

- Supplement 200mcg of chromium a day.

- People with symptoms of dysglycemia should consider supplementing 90mg Co-enzyme Q10 and 100mg lipoic acid a day.

SEVENTEEN

UNRAVELLING THE RIDDLE OF CHRONIC FATIGUE SYNDROME

Chronic fatigue syndrome, formerly known as ME, Epstein Barr, yuppie flu and by numerous other spurious titles, is a classic syndrome of symptoms that don't fit into any conventional medical model. With no real method of diagnosis or treatment, many sufferers have been told it's all in the mind and been prescribed antidepressants. Yet chronic fatigue, multiple allergies, frequent headaches, sensitivity to chemicals and environmental pollutants, chronic digestive problems, muscle aches, autism, schizophrenia, drug reactions and Gulf War syndrome are just some of the conditions that can be caused by a breakdown in the body's detoxifying mechanisms.

These mechanisms, mainly situated in the liver, kidney and brain, are a complex set of chemical processes or pathways that have the ability to recycle toxic chemicals and turn them into harmless ones; the process is known as biotransformation. Each pathway consists of a series of enzyme reactions, and each enzyme is dependent on a number of nutrients that, step by step, make our internal world safe to live in.

The detox pathways have two main phases. The first phase doesn't always result in non-toxic substances. In fact, it can produce substances which are even more poisonous. Alcohol, for example, is turned into a toxin which causes the symptoms of a hangover. Provided Phase 1 has worked well, however, Phase 2 turns these halfway products, known as intermediate metabolites, into safe substances that can be excreted from the body via the kidneys, in urine. If either phase is malfunctioning, toxins build up in the liver, kidneys and brain. This is why, for example, a person with chronic fatigue syndrome feels worse after exercise. The normal breakdown of sugar to energy doesn't work properly; instead, toxins are generated which cause muscle ache, brain fatigue and other unpleasant symptoms. Similarly, the more such people eat the more toxins their body creates.

Decreasing Your Toxic Load

Sugar is one example of how normally non-toxic nutrients become toxic if the body's detoxifying processes are out of balance. Drinking alcohol, smoking cigarettes, eating fried food, eating too much, taking drugs including paracetamol, taking in pesticide residues, breathing in pollution – these are some of the more obvious ways of overloading the body with toxins.

Normally healthy foods can also become toxins to the body if they are not digested or absorbed properly. We are designed to digest our food into simple molecules that can readily pass through the digestive tract and into the bloodstream. However, if a person doesn't digest their food properly, or if the gut wall becomes leaky, incompletely digested foods can enter unheeded into the blood. There they are likely to trigger immune 'scout' cells which treat them as invaders. The ensuing battle results in a complex of chemicals that are themselves toxins and need to be cleaned up to be safe.

The gut wall can become leaky for a number of reasons: alcohol and aspirin irritate the gut lining, as does a protein called gluten found in wheat; a deficiency of cell-building nutrients, like vitamin A, zinc, protein and essential fats, can result in a poor gut-wall structure; an overgrowth of the wrong bacteria or fungi, such as *Candida albicans*, can burrow into the intestinal wall, irritating it and causing increased permeability. Once the gut wall is permeable, perfectly normal foods can become toxic to the body.

Testing Your Detox Potential

Fortunately, modern medicine has developed non-invasive ways to test if your gut is leaky, and how well your body carries out each phase of detoxification. The gut permeability test involves drinking a fluid which contains molecules of different sizes. The degree of leakiness is then established by analysing the urine to detect which molecules have passed through the gut wall. You can also assess your liver's detoxification potential in a test which involves drinking two substances. Again, through identifying what appears in the urine when it is chemically analysed the test can show how well each phase of liver detoxification is working. These tests are available through doctors and nutrition consultants.

As well as testing your chemistry there's nothing better than testing how you feel. To this effect Dr Jeffrey Bland developed the Metabolic Screening Questionnaire, with common symptoms that indicate a low detox potential. I've produced an abbreviated checklist here. By seeing which symptoms apply to you you can get a reasonable idea of whether or not your metabolism is up to scratch.

CHECK OUT YOUR DETOX POTENTIAL

Score **1** for every symptom you have occasionally, and **2** for those you have frequently

Head ☐ Headaches, faintness, dizziness, insomnia

Eyes ☐ Watery or itchy eyes; swollen, red or sticky eyelids; bags or dark circles; blurred vision

Ears ☐ Itchy ears, earache, ear infection, drainage from ear, ringing in ears, hearing loss

Nose ☐ Stuffy nose, sinus problems, hay fever, sneezing attacks, excessive mucus formation

Mouth ☐ Chronic coughing; gagging; frequent need to clear throat; hoarseness; loss of voice; swollen or discoloured tongue, gums or lips; mouth ulcers

Skin ☐ Acne, hives, rashes, dry skin, hair loss, flushing or hot flashes, excessive sweating

Heart ☐ Irregular or skipped heartbeat, rapid or pounding heartbeat, chest pain

Lungs ☐ Chest congestion, asthma, bronchitis, shortness of breath, difficulty in breathing

Digestion ☐ Nausea or vomiting, diarrhoea, constipation, bloated feeling, belching, passing gas, heartburn, intestinal/stomach pain

Joints/ Muscles ☐ Joint/muscle aches or pain, arthritis, stiffness or limitation of movement, feeling of weakness or tiredness

Weight ☐ Binge eating/drinking, craving certain foods, excessive weight, compulsive eating, water retention, underweight

Energy ☐ Fatigue, sluggishness, apathy, lethargy, hyperactivity, restlessness

Mind ☐ Poor memory, confusion, poor comprehension, poor concentration, poor physical coordination, difficulty in making decisions, stuttering or stammering, slurred speech, learning disabilities

Emotions   ☐   Mood swings, anxiety, fear, nervousness, anger, irritability, aggressiveness, depression

TOTAL SCORE ☐

If your total score is above **25**, suspect a detox problem and clean up your diet.

If your total score is above **50**, your detox potential is under par.

If your total score is above **75,** you would be well advised to seek the help of a practitioner.

Healing the Gut

While many substances such as pesticides, food additives and alcohol are toxins in their own right, many ordinary foods become toxins if they're not properly digested and absorbed. So before you can begin detoxifying it's necessary to heal your gut. Traditionally, practitioners recommend a 'clean' diet free from toxins, plus supplemental digestive enzymes. If the gut wall is leaky, there are specific nutrients that can help to restore the balance. Supplementing beneficial bacteria, plus butyric acid and FOS (fructo-oligosaccharides), helps to normalise gut flora. Quercitin, ginkgo biloba and antioxidants such as vitamins A and C help to reduce damage, while l-glutamine, zinc and glucosamine help to heal the gut. Once that's all done, you're ready to boost your detox metabolism.

How to Detox and Boost Your Metabolism

Detoxification in the liver takes place in two phases. 'Phase 1 (oxidation) involves the activity of a super family of enzymes known as P450s, which activate a fat-soluble toxin and make it more able to be dissolved in bodily fluids, especially water,' says Jeffrey Bland. The nutrients that are needed to support a healthy Phase 1 detoxification are vitamins B2, B3, B6 and B12, folic acid, glutathione, branched chain amino acids, flavonoids and phospholipids, plus a good supply of antioxidant nutrients to disarm dangerous intermediary oxidants created during this phase.

In some people Phase 1 works really well and Phase 2 does not – in other words highly toxic free radicals are produced but not dealt with. Such people are classified as 'pathological detoxifiers' and tend to feel worse

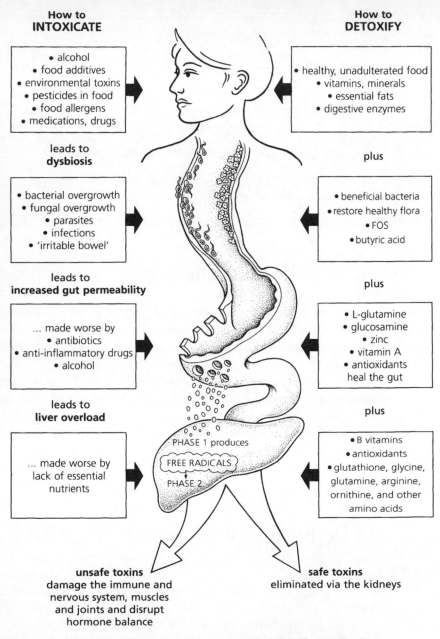

**How to
INTOXICATE**

- alcohol
- food additives
- environmental toxins
- pesticides in food
- food allergens
- medications, drugs

**leads to
dysbiosis**

- bacterial overgrowth
- fungal overgrowth
- parasites
- infections
- 'irritable bowel'

**leads to
increased gut permeability**

... made worse by
- antibiotics
- anti-inflammatory drugs
- alcohol

**leads to
liver overload**

... made worse by
lack of essential
nutrients

**How to
DETOXIFY**

- healthy, unadulterated food
- vitamins, minerals
- essential fats
- digestive enzymes

plus

- beneficial bacteria
- restore healthy flora
- FOS
- butyric acid

plus

- L-glutamine
- glucosamine
- zinc
- vitamin A
- antioxidants
heal the gut

plus

- B vitamins
- antioxidants
- glutathione, glycine,
glutamine, arginine,
ornithine, and other
amino acids

PHASE 1 produces

FREE RADICALS

PHASE 2

unsafe toxins
damage the immune and
nervous system, muscles
and joints and disrupt
hormone balance

safe toxins
eliminated via the kidneys

Fig. 10   How to intoxicate and detoxify the body

when put on a supplement programme. In such cases a liver detox test is essential.

Phase 2 of detoxification, also known as conjugation, can be stimulated into action by a specific list of nutrients including the amino acids glycine, taurine, glutamine, arginine and alanine. Cysteine, N-acetyl cysteine and methionine are also precursors for these nutrients (that is, the body can convert these two into the others).

A combination of these nutrients, and a diet which decreases the toxic load, can make an extraordinary difference to your health in a matter of weeks if not days. Fortunately, you don't have to take hundreds of supplements. Bland's team developed a special powder called Ultra Clear, which you drink as a 'shake' twice a day for two to four weeks to restore proper detoxification. There's also a product for those with a leaky gut and for the 'pathological detoxifiers' whose Phase 1 works well but whose Phase 2 has packed up. Other leading-edge nutritional companies also produce combination supplements and regimes for achieving the same goal.

In the hands of a good practitioner armed with test results, the whole process of restoring the health of the digestive tract, rebalancing the liver and detoxifying the body can be completed in three months. The results, in those who have been ill with 'untreatable', long-term chronic fatigue, are often spectacular.

Oxygen – Are You Getting Enough?

New Zealand scientist Dr Les Simpson believes he too may have found an important missing link in the understanding of chronic fatigue syndrome and muscle pain – a lack of oxygen. Oxygen is required by all cells for metabolism. It is carried around the body by red blood cells, which, when they are in the tiny blood capillaries, release the oxygen so it can pass through the capillary walls into the cells. At the capillary-cell interface the cell receives oxygen and nutrients from the blood, and at the same time gives off carbon dioxide and other unwanted by-products of metabolism.

These capillaries are only 4 microns (a millionth of a metre) wide, yet red blood cells are typically 8 microns in diameter. How, wondered Simpson, do they pass along such a narrow space? The answer is they squeeze through. Yet sometimes red blood cells are too large, while others are too inflexible and some clump together. These can create a 'log-jam' which results in a poor oxygen supply to cells, resulting in a build-up of lactic acid and poor cell function. One tell-tale sign of chronic fatigue is muscle pain after exertion. The symptoms of muscle pain also occur in polymyalgia, an increasingly common diagnosis particularly among older women. A number of researchers have also observed a lack of oxygen in the frontal lobes of the brain in people diagnosed with schizophrenia.

So what's the cure? A lack of vitamin B12 is the most common cause of over-sized red blood cells, while a lack of essential fatty acids makes them too rigid and unable to squeeze through. Niacin (vitamin B3) also helps by increasing the electrochemical charge on cells so that they repel each other and don't clump together, as well as dilating blood vessels through the release of histamine (which causes a short-term blushing effect). If this problem is suspected, it can be corrected by supplementing 100mg or more of niacin twice a day, essential fats GLA (omega-6) and EPA (omega-3) and B12.

The Energy Equation

If you tire easily it doesn't necessarily mean you have a lack of oxygen or a poor ability to detoxify. These are common contributors to chronic fatigue syndrome, which, at its worst, can leave the sufferer completely unable to function. At the other end of the spectrum, however, is tiredness, which is evidently a widespread health problem. In a survey by the Institute of Optimum Nutrition (ION), published in 1987 in a report called *The Vitamin Controversy*, 58 per cent of people complained of frequently feeling tired – a condition that can have many much simpler causes.

Researchers at ION found that, by simply improving diet and supplementing the many key vitamins and minerals needed to turn food into energy, 73 per cent of people experienced a definite improvement in energy. This strongly suggests that, for many people, the underlying cause of fatigue is more simply a lack of the right nutrients. Other factors known to contribute to tiredness are blood sugar imbalances (see Chapter 17), excessive use of stimulants such as tea and coffee, excessive use of alcohol and not enough sleep.

EIGHTEEN

THE SCIENCE OF PROLONGEVITY

Ageing is the best example of the way our genes interact with our environment to adapt to health – it is quite simply the process of becoming increasingly unable to deal with the environment. According to Professor Denham Harman from the University of Nebraska Medical School, the 'chances are 99 per cent that free radicals are the basis for ageing'. These oxidants, produced by the body every time we turn glucose into energy, eventually kill us. If we take in more oxidants, by smoking or living in a polluted city for example, and consume few antioxidants from fruit and vegetables, we age even more quickly.

To make energy we need glucose plus oxygen. Roughly a trillion molecules of oxygen are processed by each cell of the body each day. The free radicals generated produce around a hundred thousand wounds to the cell's DNA, which contains its genes. Antioxidants and the immune system repair 99 per cent of the damage, but what is left accumulates. According to geneticist Bruce Ames from the University of California at Berkeley, 'By the time you're old, we find a few million oxygen lesions per cell.' What's more, we do seem to be programed for obsolescence. Once men and women have passed their primary reproductive years, their ability to repair DNA damage declines and indeed, there is a strong association between a species' ability to repair DNA damage and its lifespan. The lost ability to repair DNA is essentially a lost ability to adapt to our environment.

So, come the age of fifty, unless you take positive steps to prevent it your body will age rapidly. That's the bad news. The good news is that almost all scientists specialising in ageing (gerontologists) now agree that simple ways already exist to add at least ten, if not twenty years to your healthy lifespan. Here's what the experts say:

> Ultimately we are going to be able to get people to live a lot longer than anyone thinks.
>
> *Dr Bruce Ames, University of California researcher and geneticist*

We could add an extra twelve to eighteen years to our lives by taking 3000-12,000mg of vitamin C a day.

Dr Linus Pauling, twice Nobel Prize winner

The evidence suggests that one can add significant years to life and obvious life to years!

Dr Emanuel Cheraskin, Emeritus Professor Of Medicine, University of Alabama

Provided you are not in the grip of degenerative disease already, you are likely to get at least a decade of vigorous years, and perhaps a lot more, no matter what age you are now [through optimal nutrition].

Dr Michael Colgan, Colgan Institute

It seems fairly certain that maximum lifespan could already be prolonged to 130 or 140 years by the exercise of very stringent measures.

Dr Roy Walford, Professor of Gerontology, UCLA

Well-rounded nutrition, including generous amounts of vitamins C and E, can contribute materially to extending the lifespan of those who are already middle aged.

Dr Roger Williams, University of Austin, Texas

'Some scientists have adopted a "wait and see" attitude,' says Professor Roy Walford. 'Of course, if they wait too long, they won't see.' The same applies to you. Do you want to apply what has been learnt about the science of pro-longevity, and reap the rewards in this life, or sit on the fence and fall off it prematurely?

Lifespan Predictions

While the average age of death in the West is currently seventy-four, geron-tologists are now predicting that a lifespan of 120 is probably achievable pro-vided you pursue an anti-ageing strategy such as the one explained here. Indeed, the longevity record is currently held by Madame Jeanne Calmant, who died in 1997 at the age of 122. To achieve a lifespan of 100, already more than twenty years on top of the average, is certainly a realistic goal. And we are not talking here of extending years of decrepitude, but rather slowing down the whole ageing process and extending your healthy lifespan. The cost of pursuing such an anti-ageing strategy is marginal when com-pared to the cost of managing ill health in the last decade of life. So here's how to do it.

Four Steps to Prolongevity

The ageing process can be slowed down in four basic steps, which are also synonymous with reducing your risk of other conditions such as cancer, heart disease, Alzheimer's, cataracts, diabetes, arthritis and infectious diseases.

Minimise your exposure to free radicals

This means:

- not smoking or being in smoky atmospheres
- reducing your exposure to pollution by cutting down on time spent in traffic jams and not living in central city areas
- steaming foods rather than frying them
- cutting down on saturated fat, found in meat, eggs and dairy products
- using cold-pressed seed oils, eating them cold (in salad dressings and spreads) and never heating them
- avoiding burnt or browned food, especially crispy cheese on the top of savoury dishes
- minimising exposure to strong sunlight and protecting yourself with a sun block

Of course, you may not want or be able to achieve this overnight. But it isn't as hard as it sounds. I live in a city, but bought a house next to a park and a river, not next to a busy road. It's sixty seconds' walk from the Institute where I teach; otherwise I work from home, thus minimising pollution. I used to love cheese on toast, but have adapted to not having it. I even eat my toast warm, not browned. It tastes fine. Instead of frying I 'steam-fry', adding a watery-based sauce to a hot pan of foods and steaming them in the herbs and spices I use to flavour each dish. I used to love getting tanned, but now enjoy the sun and protect myself at the same time. These sacrifices are a small price to pay for twenty extra years of healthy living.

Choose foods rich in antioxidants

Overall, this means:

- eating lots of fruit and vegetables, preferably organic.

A good guideline is at least five servings of fruit or vegetables a day – for example, three pieces of fruit, a salad at lunchtime and a vegetable-based dinner. There are, however, foods that are particularly rich in the key anti-ageing antioxidant nutrients. These are shown overleaf. Foods with a total score of 2 or more are the best all-rounders. If three-quarters of what you eat consists of these foods you're on the right track for a long and healthy life.

Best Foods for Antioxidants

Food	Total Score	Beta Carotene	Vitamin C	Vitamin E	Glutathione or Cysteine
		Antioxidant			
Salmon	3			✓	
Mackerel	3			✓	
Tuna	3			✓	
Nuts	3			✓	
Seeds	3			✓	
Berries	3	✓	✓		
Broccoli	3	✓	✓		
Peas	3		✓	✓	
Sweet potato	3	✓	✓	✓	
Tomatoes	3	✓	✓		
Watermelon	3	✓	✓		✓
Wheatgerm	3			✓	
Asparagus	2				✓
Avocado	2			✓	✓
Brazil nuts	2			✓	
Cabbage	2	✓			
Carrots	2	✓	✓		
Cauliflower	2		✓		
Fish	2			✓	
Garlic	2				✓
Peppers	2		✓		
Spinach	2	✓			
Watercress	2	✓	✓		
Apricots	1	✓			
Broad beans	1				
Brussels sprouts	1				
Butternut squash	1	✓			
Citrus fruit	1		✓		
Ginger	1				
Grapes	1				
Lentils + beans	1				
Mushrooms	1				
Pinenuts	1				
Soya products	1				
Wholegrains	1				

Antioxidant

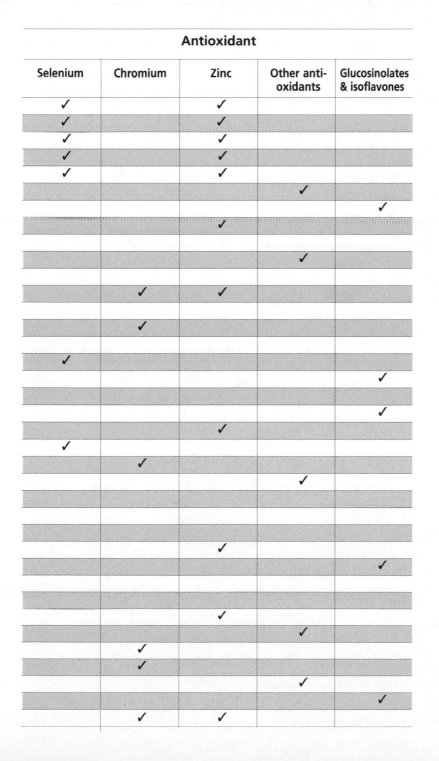

Selenium	Chromium	Zinc	Other anti-oxidants	Glucosinolates & isoflavones
✓		✓		
✓		✓		
✓		✓		
✓		✓		
✓		✓		
			✓	
				✓
		✓		
			✓	
	✓	✓		
	✓			
✓				
				✓
				✓
		✓		
✓				
	✓			
			✓	
		✓		
				✓
		✓		
			✓	
	✓			
	✓			
			✓	
				✓
	✓	✓		

Supplement antioxidants

The evidence is unequivocal that, in addition to eating a diet rich in anti-oxidants, extra supplements further increase your chances of extending your healthy lifespan. The key nutrients are shown below, together with the ideal daily intake. In building your supplement programme start with a good, high-potency multivitamin and mineral and then add extra accordingly. In addition, every day I take two high-potency comprehensive antioxidant supplements and two 1g vitamin C tablets. That adequately covers the nutrients listed below.

- **Vitamin A** 7500ius (2250mcg) a day. This powerful, fat-based antioxidant protects against lung cancer and helps keep cell membranes strong in the face of free radical attack. A certain amount of betacarotene is converted into vitamin A; however, it's good to have a direct source of vitamin A, which is found in meat and fish.

- **Betacarotene** 7–15mg a day. That's equivalent to between 12,500ius (3800mcgRE) and 50,000ius (15,000mcgRE). These higher levels may not be necessary if your diet provides significant quantities. For example, a glass of carrot juice can give you 25mg. Once again, betacarotene stops cancer, prevents heart attacks, boosts the immune system and slows down ageing.

- **Vitamin C** 2–5g a day. Start with 2g (2000mg) and add 1g for every decade over the age of forty. There are two schools of thought on vitamin C: those who say 500–1000mg is optimal, and those, like Linus Pauling, who note that animals produce the equivalent of 1–16g a day and there-fore advocate larger quantities. But even 300mg a day can add six years to a man's life, according to research by UCLA's James Enstrom.[112] Higher levels have proved to give immunity a boost and to protect against cancer.

- **Vitamin E** 400ius a day. This is the most important antioxidant protector for fats in the body. Numerous studies have shown that supplementation halves the risk of cardiovascular disease. It also improves immunity.

- **Co-enzyme Q10** 30–90mg a day. This is an antioxidant within mito-chondria, the cells' energy factories. Although it is not classified as an essential nutrient, many gerontologists now supplement it. Fat-soluble forms are the best absorbed.

- **Zinc** 15–30mg a day. Zinc is the most commonly deficient mineral – most people get less than 8mg a day. It's an antioxidant and a key immune system booster and needs to be increased with age.

- **Chromium** 200mcg a day. Chromium's major protective role is in preventing dysglycemia and Syndrome X. Once sugar balance is lost, glucose becomes a major oxidant in the body, damaging proteins.

- **Calcium and magnesium** 500mg and 300mg a day respectively. Ideal needs are more like 1000mg and 500mg respectively, but as long as you're eating some seeds, nuts and plenty of vegetables these levels represent a top-up to optimal anti-ageing levels.

- **Glutathione, cysteine and glutamine** 500mg a day. Glutahione is a key antioxidant within cells and helps the body to detoxify toxins. It is part of the antioxidant enzyme glutathione peroxidase, which is co-dependent on selenium. You can make glutathione in the body, a process stimulated by vitamin C, eating vegetables such as broccoli, cabbage and Brussels sprouts, and supplementing glutamine. From cysteine, which is easier for the body to absorb and deliver to cells, you can make glutathione. The best forms to supplement are either reduced glutathione, N-acetyl-cysteine or, indeed, glutamine. A total of 500mg of these represents a top-up on dietary sources.

- **Selenium** 100–200mcg a day. Once again, this potent antioxidant protects against cancer and heart disease and boosts immunity. People's dietary intakes are rarely above 50mcg a day, hence the need for supplementation.

- **Genistein and diadzein** 100–200mg a day. You won't find these in many supplements, as they are very 'state of the art'. They are present in soya produce, and regulate hormone levels as well as protecting against cancer. A 300ml (just over ½ pint) portion of soya milk provides 100mg of each of these phytonutrients as does a 100mg serving of tofu.

Cut down on calories

Calorie restriction is not the same as malnutrition – it's about giving the body exactly what it needs and no more. Many foods in our typical modern diet provide 'empty' calories. That is, they provide sugar or saturated fat, but none of the micronutrients needed to process them. These foods are out if you want to extend your lifespan. Nutrient-dense foods such as organic carrots, apples, nuts and seeds provide as many nutrients as calories, plus, in the case of fresh fruit and vegetables, plenty of essential and calorie-free water. The leaner you are, the longer you are likely to live.

One proven way to extend lifespan is to eat less. Since the first animal experiments in 1935, studies on several species have shown that animals which eat 30–40 per cent fewer calories extend their lifespan by a third to a half. However, it isn't just a question of limiting calories. These animals were given optimum nutrition as well as fewer calories, with good intakes of antioxidants. There's every reason to assume the same principle applies to humans. Consider the islanders of Okinawa in Japan. They eat 17–40 per cent fewer calories than other Japanese and have more centenarians than any other population. According to Dr Roy Walford of UCLA Medical School, 'You can even extend longevity by restricting food even after full adulthood and middle age.'

Having a high-quality diet with minimal calories means less work for the body. You are giving yourself exactly what you need and no more. But how much less do you need to eat? Walford says that you can extend your lifespan by cutting your calories by 10–25 per cent. He eats between 1500 and 2000 calories a day, compared to the average intake of 2500 calories for a woman and 3000 for a man.

One way to restrict calories is simply to eat less. Another is to fast or have a modified fast one day a week. This may mean, for example, just eating fruit. I keep my overall calorie intake low by eating a substantial breakfast and dinner, but a small lunch or sometimes no lunch and snacking on fruit throughout the day. Life insurance companies are well aware of the correlation between weight and longevity. Standard weight charts give an ideal weight range for your height. Generally, the ideal weight for increased life expectancy is at the low end of this range. What really counts is keeping your body fat percentage down, which can also be helped by regular exercise. This is the percentage of your body that is fat. Ideal levels are 15–25 per cent for a woman and 12–20 per cent for a man.

PART 5

ENVIRONMENTAL MEDICINE

Good planets are hard to find.

NINETEEN

THE ART OF CHEMICAL SELF-DEFENCE

It isn't just what you do eat that makes a difference to your health. It's what you don't eat. Nowadays, the average person eats in a year 5kg (12lb) of food additives and has 4.5 litres (a gallon) of pesticides and herbicides sprayed on the fruit and vegetables they eat. They also consume nitrates, hormone and antibiotic residues, lead, aluminium and numerous other undesirable substances both from water and food. Six thousand new chemicals have been introduced into our food, our homes and the world around us in the last twenty years. These and other pollutants add to the burden our bodies already have to cope with from self-selected harmful substances including alcohol, cigarettes, free radicals in fried food, methylxanthines in coffee, and a host of naturally occurring toxins present in small amounts even in healthy food. The proliferation of food pollution has led to a new science – the science of 'antinutrition'.

First coined by Professor Bryce-Smith, a chemist from Reading University who alerted us to the dangers of lead in petrol back in 1983, the term 'antinutrient' is defined as any substance that prevents the absorption, interferes with the action, or promotes the loss of a nutrient, for example a vitamin or mineral. Most of the substances we think of as bad for us are bad precisely because they interfere with the vital functions of essential nutrients:

- **Lead** affects intelligence and behaviour by interfering with **calcium and zinc**, both needed for normal brain function

- **Coffee** interferes with **iron** absorption, rendering less than a third of the iron taken in available for use in the body

- **Burnt or fried food** destroys **vitamins C and E**, as does **smoking**

- **Alcohol** destroys **B vitamins** and renders most **minerals** less available

- **Refined sugar** causes a loss of **chromium**

- **Refined** flour is disproportionately high in cadmium, which robs the body of **zinc** (and is therefore known as a zinc antagonist)

- **Aluminium**, in widespread use for food packaging is another **zinc** antagonist

- **Acid rain** renders **minerals** in the soil less absorbable

There is no doubt that the nutritionist of the twenty-first century will be as heavily involved in advising people what to avoid as in advising people what to eat for health.

Some scientists, often employed by the industries that generate pollution, argue that antinutrients are present in natural foods, which is true, and there's no need to be alarmed. But nature has a knack of putting the good with the bad to give us protection. The coffee bean is a stimulant, but the fruit, the coffee berry, is a relaxant. Soya beans are high in aluminium, but also in zinc. Wheat is high in cadmium, but the bran is high in zinc; once flour is refined, though, the protective zinc is removed, leaving an excess of cadmium.

There is no doubt that most food pollution is the direct result of mankind messing around with natural foods for the sake of profit or convenience.

- **Nitrates**, for example, have been used for years to speed up the growth of plants for increased profit. The excessive use of nitrates has poisoned both our food and water: in the body they combine with amines to produce cancer-forming nitrosamines.

- **Growth hormones**, coupled with **high-protein diets**, are given to animals to speed up meat formation. These hormones in turn disrupt the hormone balance of those eating the meat, increasing their risk for cancer.

- **Aluminium** is a material widely used in food packaging, despite the fact that excess aluminium is clearly associated with premature senility and memory loss. Aluminium is also found in antacid medication, saucepans and toothpaste, and is added to many water supplies as part of the 'cleansing' process!

- **Essential fats** are removed from foods because they go off, and **hydrogenated fats** are added, despite the fact that a high consumption of saturated and hydrogenated fats is associated with an increased risk of heart disease, cancer and inflammatory diseases.

Although humans are equipped with clever mechanisms for detoxifying many harmful substances, in many of us these mechanisms are becoming increasingly overloaded. When this happens, toxins are laid down in bone, fat, brain and other tissue. When calcium is released for muscle activity, so are toxins. When fat is used for energy, yet more are released. These toxins ultimately affect our brain, nervous system, liver, kidneys and other vital organs.

The effects of pollution are cumulative, and rarely seen at the time the pollution occurs. It is therefore not easy to make a cause-and-effect link in pollution-related diseases, when you consider that the pollution may have been slight over several years, or may have occurred decades earlier. In addition, most diseases have a number of origins. We can be pretty certain of many links, though:

- Increased toxic metal exposure (predominantly lead and cadmium) causes a measurable decline in intelligence, performance and behaviour in children, and an increased risk for birth defects and low-weight babies

- The level of nitrites and nitrates in most water supplies, especially in rural areas, may increase the risk of certain forms of cancer

- Long-term ingestion of small amounts of aluminium from cooking utensils and food packaging is associated with premature senility

- The widespread use of pesticides increases the incidence of immune-related diseases

- The level of free oxidising radicals, from our polluted air, from fried and processed foods, from passive smoking and from exhaust fumes, coupled with a deficiency in antioxidant nutrients, increases our risk of most forms of cancer and heart disease

- Exposure to plastic residues disrupts hormone balance, exacerbating menopausal problems in men and women, increasing the risk of hormone-related cancer and disturbing sexual programming during foetal development

These alarming facts represent just the tip of the iceberg. Other diseases that have been associated with a high level of pollutants include:

- all forms of arthritis
- allergies
- candidiasis
- chronic fatigue syndrome
- repeated infections
- hyperactivity
- high blood pressure
- asthma
- acne
- eczema
- schizophrenia

'Minor' symptoms associated with increased body burden of pollutants include:

- lethargy
- drowsiness
- mood swings
- inability to concentrate
- intolerance of fat or alcohol
- poor skin
- body odour
- headaches
- nausea
- skin rashes
- frequent infections
- multiple allergies

All these symptoms can occur for other reasons, such as specific diseases or lack of certain essential nutrients. But even when these are the result of increased body pollution, they are far more likely to occur in people who are not adequately nourished. This is because most pollutants do their damage by interfering with the body's ability to make good use of nutrients. What's more, the body's detoxifying mechanisms are themselves greatly enhanced by an optimum intake of essential nutrients, including vitamins, minerals, essential fatty acids and protein.

Pollution Solutions

So how do you protect yourself from pollution? The first step is to reduce your intake of pollutants. If by now you're suffering from 'acute pollution paranoia', console yourself with the fact that you cannot avoid all pollution. Harmful substances have always existed, even within foods whose overall effect on the body is definitely positive. The best you can do is keep your overall exposure down as far as possible. One way to do this is by increasing your dietary intake of certain factors that minimise the absorption of pollutants. For example, when vitamin C is present nitrites are less likely to form cancer-producing nitrosamines in the digestive tract.

The second step is to boost your natural detoxifying mechanisms. This can be done by improving your diet and taking protective vitamin and mineral supplements. So let's now look at the major pollutants, ways of avoiding or reducing our exposure to them, and ways of protecting ourselves from their harmful effects.

Lead and Other Toxic Elements

The most common toxic metals are lead, aluminium, cadmium, copper and mercury. We take in lead from air, food and water, but the main source is exhaust fumes, although levels are diminishing as more and more cars become lead-free. The lead in exhaust fumes ends up in the soil and on the plants we eat. There is nowhere in Britain that is not contaminated with lead. Even the levels in Greenland ice are a thousand times higher now than a hundred years ago [113] Smokers are particularly likely to have high cadmium levels.

Avoidance

- Avoid buying unwrapped fruit and vegetables that do not require peeling and have been exposed to street traffic.

- Wash all fruit and vegetables, preferably in a bowl of water with two table-spoons of vinegar added. This acidifies the water and helps remove heavy metals.

- Discard the outer leaves of cabbage, lettuce etc.

- Be wary of eating fish caught off the British coast. It is said that frozen fish is caught in the further reaches of the North Sea and Arctic Ocean. Limit your fish intake when you don't know the source, and certainly avoid local shellfish or a Dover sole from Dover.

- Don't smoke and, where possible, avoid passive smoking.

- Minimise the amounts of food you eat that is packaged in aluminium. Don't grill food on, or wrap food in, aluminium foil.

- Don't take antacid medication containing aluminium.

- Don't use aluminium pots and pans. Many non-stick pans are aluminium once you've worn through the non-stick bit, which incidentally is toxic.

- Drink bottled water or invest in a water filter, especially if your water pipes are copper and you live in a soft water area.

Protection

- Make sure your diet provides plenty of calcium, zinc and vitamin C, which are heavy metal antagonists. That means eating lots of nuts, seeds, green leafy vegetables, wheatgerm, fresh fruit etc.

- Eat foods high in pectin, which is also protective. Such foods include apples, bananas and carrots.

- Minimise your consumption of alcohol, which increases the absorption of lead.

- Supplement your diet daily with at least 1000mg of vitamin C, 200mg of calcium and 10mg of zinc. Double this amount if you live in a city.

Nitrates

Governments and the World Health Organisation have known for many years that nitrates and nitrites are toxic and in 1970 they set limits for water and food levels. Once inside the body nitrates combine with amines, present in almost all foods, to form nitrosamines, which are highly carcinogenic compounds. Most water authorities in Britain do not have the necessary purification equipment and have stated that millions of people are consuming water containing levels of nitrates above the EU top limit. The problem is especially severe in arable areas and the Thames basin, where nitrates, originating from use in fertilisers, have filtered down into the water table. The only way to solve this problem is for farmers to stop using nitrate-based fertilisers and switch to organic methods.

As well as the problem with water, vegetables grown with nitrate-based fertilisers can be high in nitrates. These chemicals are also added to cured meats such as ham, sausages, bacon and pies. Of our total intake, 70 per cent comes from vegetables, 21 per cent from water and 6 per cent from meat.

Avoidance

- Drink filtered or bottled water.

- Eat organically grown produce wherever possible.

- Brush and floss your teeth regularly. It is estimated that up to 65 per cent of nitrites absorbed are produced in the mouth by bacteria.

- Avoid foods that include nitrates or nitrites as preservatives, which includes many meat products.

- Make sure your protein intake is adequate but not excessive.

Protection

- To inhibit nitrosamine formation, supplement your diet with at least 1000mg of vitamin C a day. The ideal way is to take some vitamin C with each main meal.

Pesticides

With today's chemical farming, even the old adage that 'an apple a day keeps the doctor away' must be questioned. For the caterpillar, one brief journey across the average apple is enough to kill it. But what about us? According to the World Health Organisation, there were 3 million cases of severe pesticide poisoning and twenty thousand deaths globally in 1996. In the UK there are at least five thousand suspected pesticide poisoning incidents annually, with some seven hundred victims, including five hundred children under the age of ten, admitted to hospital.

A survey by the Ministry of Agriculture (see p. 128) found that 89–99 per cent of all fresh fruit, cereals and vegetables are sprayed with pesticides. Some of these are used for animal feed, which means that most meat and milk is also contaminated by pesticides. Although few proper surveys have been carried out to discover the extent of the problem, the Association for Public Analysts is gravely concerned. When its scientists randomly tested 305 fruits, 31 samples contained pesticide residues above the safety levels, while a further 72 samples showed lower pesticide residues. Some fruits, particularly strawberries, raspberries, grapes and tomatoes, had measurable levels of at least six different pesticides! More recent scares have concerned the level of chemicals in carrots and lettuce. In 1994, a survey by the Ministry of Agriculture, Fisheries and Food (MAFF) of carrots found some to have levels 25 times higher than the safety limit. In 1995, 10 per cent of lettuces tested had levels in excess of the safety limit.

But food isn't the only way we take in pesticides. The use of pesticides is so widespread that they even make their way into water supplies. The UK government sets Maximum Admissible Concentrations (MACs) for each pesticide and for total pesticides in water. Between June 1985 and June 1987, these levels were breached by water authorities 98 times for single pesticides, and 70 times for total pesticides. Current estimates are that 14.5 million customers consume water with pesticide levels above permissible limits.

Avoidance

- Select organic fruit and vegetables wherever possible.

- Wash or peel non-organic produce.

- Choose fruit and vegetables in season. This means that your exposure to the chemicals used to delay ripening, prolong shelf-life, preserve colour and so on will be limited.

- Drink filtered, distilled or spring water.

Protection

- Supplement your diet with antioxidant nutrients – vitamins A, C and E and the minerals zinc and selenium – since the detoxification of many pesticides involves these nutrients.

Food Additives

Numerous chemicals are purposely added to our food to change its colour, preserve it, prevent rancidity, keep fats emulsified and render foods stable. Most of them are synthetic compounds, some with known negative health effects. But more importantly, we don't really know what the long-term consequences of consuming such large amounts of additives are.

Avoidance

- Avoid all foods containing additives. A few notable exceptions are listed below.

Good Additives

Colours	E101 (vitamin B2)
	E160 (carotene, vitamin A)
Antioxidants	E300–304 (vitamin C)
	E306–309 (tocopherols, such as vitamin E)
Emulsifiers	E322 (lecithin)
Stabilisers	E375 (niacin)
	E440 (pectin)

Protection

- Since foods without preservatives are more likely to go off, it's important to buy fresh produce and consume it relatively quickly.

THE TOP TWENTY ADDITIVES TO AVOID

Name	E Number	How used	What you need to know
Allura Red AC	E129	Widely used as food colouring, in snacks, sauces, preserves, soups, wine, cider etc.	Avoid if you suffer from asthma, rhinitis (including hay fever) and urticaria (an allergic rash also known as hives).
Amaranth	E123	Food colour used in wine, spirits, fish roe.	Banned in the US. Avoid if you suffer from asthma, rhinitis, urticaria and other allergies.
Aspartame	E951	Widely used as a sweetener in snacks, sweets, alcohol, desserts, 'diet' foods.	Aspartame may affect people with PKU (phenylketonuria). Recent reports show the possibility of headaches, blindness, and seizures with long-term high-dose aspartame.
Benzoic acid	E210	Widely used preservative in many foods, including drinks, low-sugar products, cereals, meat products.	Can temporarily inhibit the function of digestive enzymes and may deplete glycine levels. Should be avoided by those with allergic conditions such as hay fever, hives and asthma.

Name	E Number	How used	What you need to know
Brilliant Black BN	E151	Widely used in drinks, sauces, snacks, wines, cheese, etc.	People who suffer from allergic conditions, asthma, rhinitis, urticaria, etc, should avoid this substance.
Butylated hydroxy-anisole	E320	Very widely used as a preservative, particularly in fat-containing foods, confectionery, meats.	The International Agency For Research On Cancer say that BHA is possibly carcinogenic to humans. BHA also interacts with nitrites to form chemicals known to be mutagenic (they cause changes in the DNA of cells).
Calcium benzoate	E213	Preservative in many foods, including drinks, low-sugar products, cereals, meat products.	Can temporarily inhibit the function of digestive enzymes and may deplete levels of the amino acid glycine. Should be avoided by those with hay fever, hives and asthma.
Calcium sulphite	E226	Very widely used, mainly as a preservative in a vast array of foods – from burgers to biscuits, from frozen mushrooms to horseradish pulp.	In the US sulphites are banned from many foods, including meat, because they make old produce look fresh. They can cause bronchial problems, flushing, low-blood pressure, tingling, and anaphylactic shock. The International Labour Organisation (ILO) says avoid them if you suffer from bronchial asthma, cardiovascular or respiratory problems and emphysema.
Monosodium glutamate (MSG)	E621	Widely used as a flavouring enhancer.	Those sensitive to monosodium glutamate have felt symptoms including pressure on the head, seizures, chest pains, headache, nausea, burning sensations and tightness of face. Many baby-food producers have stopped adding MSG to their products.
Ponceau 4R, Conchineal Red A	E124	Widely used as colouring.	People who suffer from asthma, rhinitis or urticaria may find their symptoms become worse following consumption of foods containing this colouring.

Name	E Number	How used	What you need to know
Potassium benzoate	E212	See calcium benzoate (opposite).	See calcium benzoate (opposite).
Potassium nitrate	E249	Used as a preservative in cured meats and canned meat products.	Three main health concerns: it can lower the oxygen-carrying capacity of the blood; it may combine with other substances to form nitrosamines, which are carcinogenic, and it may have an atrophying effect on the adrenal gland.
Propyl p-hydroxy-benzoate, propyl-paraben, and paraben	E216	Preservatives in cereals, snacks, pâté, meat products, confectionery.	Parabens have been identified as the cause of chronic dermatitis in numerous instances.
Saccharin and its Na, K and Ca salts	E954	Very widely used sweetener, found in diet, and no-added-sugar products.	The International Agency For Research On Cancer has concluded that saccharin is possibly carcinogenic to humans.
Sodium metabisulphite	E223	Widely used as a preservative and antioxidant.	May provoke life-threatening asthma – a woman developed severe asthma after eating a salad with a vinegar-based dressing containing E223.
Sodium sulphite	E221	Preservative used in wine-making and other processed foods.	Sulphites have been associated with triggering asthma attacks. Most asthmatics are sensitive to sulphites in food.
Stannous chloride (tin)	E512	Antioxidant and colour-retention agent in canned and bottled foods, fruit juices.	Acute poisoning has been reported from ingestion of fruit juices containing concentrations of tin greater than 250mg per litre – causing nausea, vomiting, diarrhoea and headaches.
Sulphur dioxide	E220	Very widely used preservative.	Sulphur dioxide reacts with a wide range of substances found in food, including various essential vitamins, minerals, enzymes and essential fatty acids. The most common adverse reaction to sulphites is bronchial problems, particularly in those prone

Name	E Number	How used	What you need to know
Sulphur dioxide (contd)	E220		to asthma. Other adverse reactions may include hypotension (low blood pressure), flushing, tingling sensations and anaphylactic shock. The International Labour Organisation says you should avoid E220 if you suffer from conjunctivitis, bronchitis, emphysema, bronchial asthma or cardiovascular disease.
Sunset Yellow FCF, Orange Yellow S	E110	Widely used food colouring.	Some animal studies have indicated growth retardation and severe weight loss. People with asthma, rhinitis or urticaria should avoid this product.
Tartrazine	E102	Widely used yellow food colour.	May cause allergic reactions in perhaps 15 per cent of the population. It may be a cause of asthmatic attacks and has been implicated in bouts of hyperactivity disorder in children. Those who suffer from asthma, rhinitis and urticaria may find symptoms worsen after consumption.

(reproduced from *Secret Ingredients* by permission of Peter Cox and Bantam Books)

Free Radicals

The single greatest cause of ill health is probably free oxidising radicals, also known as oxidants. These are incomplete molecules containing oxygen which have an uneven electrical charge, much like a magnet. All stable atoms and collections of atoms, called molecules, have an even electrical charge but free radicals don't, so they try to complete themselves, like a wanton bachelor looking for a mate. The trouble is, in order to make themselves stable they damage neighbouring cells, generating more free radicals. This can set up a chain reaction of damage until the free radical is disarmed by an antioxidant such as vitamin C. Free radicals increase the risk of cancer and heart disease, as well as weakening the immune system.

Avoidance

- Avoid fried foods as much as possible.

- If you do fry, use olive oil or butter, never polyunsaturated oils.

- Avoid excessive exposure to strong sunlight.

- Minimise your consumption of browned or barbecued foods.

- Avoid smoking and smoky atmospheres.

- Don't eat rancid nuts or seeds.

Protection

- Supplement your diet with the antioxidant nutrients – vitamins A, C and E, selenium and zinc. All these nutrients are provided in any good anti-oxidant complex supplement.

- Exercise at least twice a week.

- Practise relaxation or meditation techniques that involve deep breathing. This helps to bring oxygen to your cells and to combat the effects of free radicals.

Pharmaceutical Drugs

The British nation's consumption of medical drugs is among the highest in the world. The UK pharmaceutical industry turns over a staggering £4.3 billion a year. But are they all necessary? The answer is no. For example, even the use of aspirin for mild pain and headaches does us no long-term good; the human body has no need for its active ingredient – salicylic acid. Continual use of aspirin is known to increase the risk of stomach ulceration and kidney disease, to block vitamin C uptake and to lower folic acid levels. Wherever possible, drugs are best avoided. However, do not stop or reduce any prescribed medication without first consulting your doctor.

Avoidance

- Avoid excessive use of painkillers.

- Avoid antacids containing aluminium.

- Avoid frequent use of antibiotics.

- Avoid anti-inflammatory drugs, both steroid-based and non-steroidal.

- Avoid the use of antidepressants and sleeping pills as much as possible.

- Investigate natural and barrier methods of birth control rather than taking the Pill.

Protection

- If you take painkillers regularly, increase your daily vitamin C intake by 1000mg.

- If you are on a course of antibiotics take a high-strength B complex during the course, and supplement beneficial bacteria (such as *acidophilus*) for two weeks after the course.

- If you are on the Pill take a high-strength B complex and extra B6 (100mg a day) plus 15mg zinc a day.

- If you take sleeping pills or antidepressants also take a high-strength B complex (if you are taking MAOI antidepressants such as Nardil or Parstelin check your B complex supplement is free of yeast, which is incompatible with this class of drug, as is alcohol).

TWENTY

ALLERGIES – ARE YOU IMMUNE?

An estimated one in three people has an allergy. Some of these are to airborne substances such as pollen (hay fever), house dust mite or cat's fur, others to chemicals in food, household products or the environment. But the most common category of allergy-provoking substances is the food you eat. In a survey of 3000 adults, 43 per cent said they experienced adverse reactions to food.[114]

If you get three or more of the symptoms shown overleaf, you probably have an allergy and most likely to something you are eating. The most common allergy-provoking foods are:

- wheat (bread, biscuits, cereals, pasta)
- dairy produce (milk, cheese, yoghurt)
- alcohol (especially beer and wine)
- coffee
- tea
- chocolate
- nuts
- eggs
- oranges
- chemical additives in food

If you eat any one of these foods two or three times a day and would find them difficult to give up, it may be worth testing to see if you're allergic to them.

What Is an Allergy?

The best-known definition of an allergy is 'any idiosyncratic reaction where the immune system is clearly involved'. The immune system, which is the body's defence system, has the ability to produce 'markers' for substances it doesn't like. The classic markers are antibodies called IgE (immunoglobulin

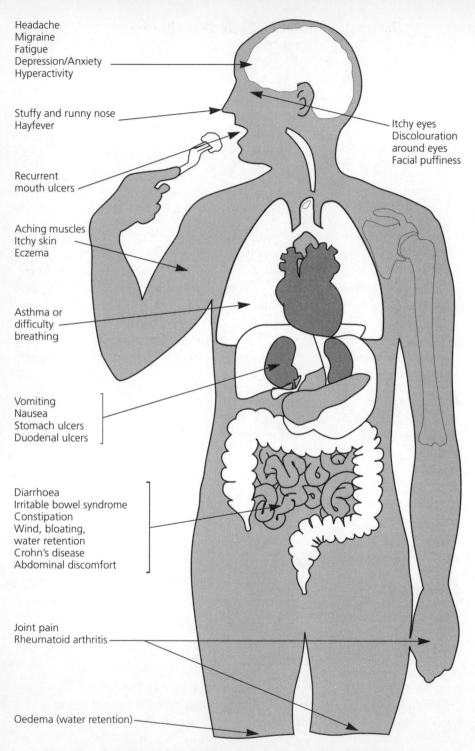

Headache
Migraine
Fatigue
Depression/Anxiety
Hyperactivity

Stuffy and runny nose
Hayfever

Recurrent
mouth ulcers

Aching muscles
Itchy skin
Eczema

Asthma or
difficulty
breathing

Vomiting
Nausea
Stomach ulcers
Duodenal ulcers

Diarrhoea
Irritable bowel syndrome
Constipation
Wind, bloating,
water retention
Crohn's disease
Abdominal discomfort

Joint pain
Rheumatoid arthritis

Oedema (water retention)

Itchy eyes
Discolouration
around eyes
Facial puffiness

Fig. 11   Symptoms associated with food allergy and intolerance

type E). These attach themselves to what are called 'mast cells' in the body. When the offending food, called an allergen, combines with its specific IgE antibody, the IgE molecule triggers the mast cell to release granules containing histamine and other chemicals that cause allergy symptoms – skin rashes, hay fever, rhinitis, sinusitis, asthma and eczema. Severe allergies to shellfish or peanuts, for example, can cause immediate gastrointestinal upsets or swelling in the face or throat. All these reactions are immediate, severe and inflammatory, and are known as Type 1 allergic reactions.

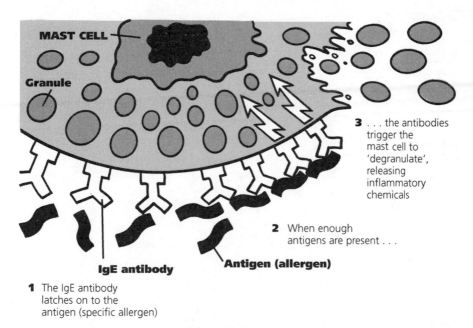

3 . . . the antibodies trigger the mast cell to 'degranulate', releasing inflammatory chemicals

2 When enough antigens are present . . .

1 The IgE antibody latches on to the antigen (specific allergen)

Fig. 12   How IgE-based allergic reactions happen

Hidden Allergies

The view emerging now is that most allergies and intolerances, diplomatically called 'idiosyncratic' reactions by some, are not IgE-based. There is a new school of thought and a new generation of allergy tests, designed to detect intolerances not based on IgE antibody reactions but probably involving another marker, known as IgG. According to Dr James Braly, director of Immuno Laboratories which developed the IgG ELISA test, 'Food allergy is not rare, nor are the effects limited to the air passages, the skin and digestive tract. Most food allergies are delayed reactions, taking anywhere from an hour to three days to show themselves, and are therefore much harder to

detect. Delayed food allergy appears to be simply the inability of your digestive tract to prevent large quantities of partially digested and undigested food
from entering the bloodstream.'

This is not a new idea. Since the 1950s pioneering allergists such as Dr
Theron Randolph, Herbert Rinkel, Dr Arthur Coca, and, more recently, Dr
William Philpott and Dr Marshall Mandel have written about delayed
sensitivities causing far-reaching effects on all systems of the body. These
scientists were the 'heretics' of classic allergy theory, but now their theories
are being proved as methods advance for determining other types of
immune reactions.

IgG antibodies were first discovered in the 1960s and are still considered
reasonably irrelevant by some conventional allergists. The problem, say the
critics, is that most people have many IgG-based reactions to foods without
apparently suffering from allergies. The IgG antibodies may serve as tags but
don't initiate a reaction. However, say the advocates, a large build-up of IgG
antibodies to a particular food indicates a chronic, long-term sensitivity or
food intolerance. Dr Hill, researching in Australia, found that the majority of
food-sensitive children reacted to foods after two or more hours. In contrast, IgE reactions are immediate, suggesting that a build-up of IgG antibodies may be a primary factor in food sensitivity.

According to Dr Jonathan Brostoff, consultant in medical immunology at
the Middlesex Hospital Medical School, certain ingested substances can
cause the release of histamine and invoke classic allergic symptoms without
involving IgE. These substances include lectins (in peanuts), shellfish, tomatoes, pork, alcohol, chocolate, pineapple, papaya, buckwheat, sunflower

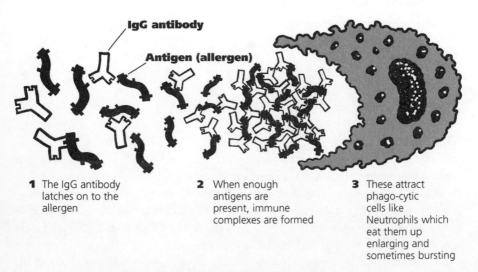

1 The IgG antibody latches on to the allergen

2 When enough antigens are present, immune complexes are formed

3 These attract phago-cytic cells like Neutrophils which eat them up enlarging and sometimes bursting

Fig. 13   How IgG-based allergic reactions happen

products, mangoes and mustard. He also thinks it is possible that undigested proteins could directly affect mast cells (which contain histamine) in the gut, causing the classic symptoms of allergy.

One common cause of allergic reactions is a substantial production of antibodies (mainly IgG) in response to an allergen in the blood. This results in large immune complexes. 'It is the sheer weight of numbers that causes a problem,' says Brostoff. 'These immune complexes are like litter going round in the bloodstream.' The litter is cleaned up by cells, principally neutrophils, that act like vacuum cleaners. Cytotoxic allergy tests are designed to measure changes in number, size and activity of neutrophils when exposed to certain foods, so as to determine possible food allergies.

How IgG and IgE antibodies relate to one another is another area of debate. Allergy specialist Dr Braly has seen a number of patients who have both an immediate and delayed reaction to a food, suggesting a link between the immediate short-term IgE-type reaction and the delayed IgG reaction. Dr Anders Hoy from Denmark suspects that long-term build-up of IgG in response to a particular food might switch to an IgE-type sensitivity, causing an immediate allergic reaction.

Why Food Allergy?

Have you ever wondered whether the food you eat actually wants to be eaten? In many cases it appears that it does not. Most forms of food try their best to protect themselves from predators – with spikes, thorns and chemical toxins. The idea that food is 'good' is far from the truth: most foods contain numerous toxins as well as beneficial nutrients. Omnivores – creatures eating both plant and animal food – like us have a high risk-high return strategy as far as food is concerned. We try different foods, and if we don't get sick then it's OK. But this short-sighted test has failed in many instances. Indeed, even today the average diet kills most people in the long-run.

Some foods are actually designed to be eaten. For example, many fruits rely on animals eating them to spread the growth of their species. The idea is that the animals, such as us human beings, eat the fruit and deposit the seed some distance from the original tree with a rich manure starter kit. However, the fruit has to protect itself from unwanted scavengers such as bacteria or fungi that simply rot the seed. The seed is often hard to crack and toxic – apricot kernels, for instance, contain cyanide compounds. For protective reasons wild food contains a massive chemical arsenal to ward off specific foes. Food and us have been fighting for survival since the beginning of time.

So why do these food intolerances occur? Are they simply a reaction to the less desirable toxins in food? The answer is unlikely to be that simple.

After all, over millions of years of evolution we have developed complex detoxification processes to protect ourselves from these chemicals. A number of theories exist, many of which have good supporting evidence.

Leaky Gut Syndrome?

The best place to start is the digestive tract, since that is where food comes into contact with us. The textbooks tell us that large food molecules get broken down into simple amino acids, fatty acids and simple sugars. Only these pass through the gut wall into the body, where they can be used as nutrients. Anything larger than these simple products of digestion is considered a foe. Could it be that undigested food or leaky gut walls could expose the immune system to food particles that trigger a reaction? This might explain why foods that are frequently eaten are more likely to cause a reaction. Indeed, recent research shows that people with food allergies do tend to have leaky gut walls.

Dr Braly suspects that many allergy sufferers may have excessively leaky gut walls, allowing undigested proteins to enter the blood and cause reactions. Consumption of alcohol, frequent use of aspirin, deficiency in essential fatty acids or a gastrointestinal infection or infestation such as candidiasis are all possible contributors to leaky gut syndrome that need to be corrected in order to reduce a person's sensitivity to foods. A lack of key nutrients such as zinc can also make the gut wall more permeable than it should be. Wheat is one of the commonest food allergens in Britain. As well as being a relatively new addition to the human diet, first being cultivated a mere ten thousand years ago, it contains a powerful intestinal irritant called gluten. In extremely sensitive or possibly less well-adapted people, the protrusions along the gut wall, called villi, through which we absorb all our nutrients, are completely destroyed by exposure to gluten. Perhaps many of us have less severe reactions.

Gut-associated Immune Reactions

Although leaky gut syndrome may be part of the reason, it is unlikely to be the whole story. Evidence is accumulating to suggest that the gut wall is far less selective than originally thought, even in healthy people. In one study, healthy adults were given potato starch – which should not normally pass through the gut wall intact – in water to drink. After fifteen to thirty minutes blood samples were taken, and found to contain up to 300 starch grains per millilitre of blood. So why weren't these people developing allergies?

The answer to this may lie in special immune cells present in patches along the digestive tract. Known as Peyer's patches, these cells sample the food you eat and desensitise the immune system so that it doesn't react to your food. It seems that most food molecules are recognisably different from undesirable toxins and harmful organisms. Perhaps some people's gut-associated immune system isn't desensitising them from the food they eat. Indeed, their immune system may even be on red alert when certain food particles arrive. The result of this is that antibodies are released which attach themselves to the allergen-forming immune complexes that encourage inflammation. As well as leading to symptoms such as bloating, abdominal pain and diarrhoea, this reaction may result in undigested food passing through the gut wall and causing immune reactions in the bloodstream, with less localised effects.

Digestive Enzymes

These problems may be particularly severe in people who don't produce enough of the right digestive enzymes, which leads to large quantities of big, undigested food molecules reaching the gut wall. One research study of people with a sensitivity to man-made chemicals showed that 90 per cent of them produced inadequate amounts of one digestive enzyme, compared to 20 per cent in a group of healthy people. Undigested food may increase the chances of a localised reaction, increase the number of large molecules entering the blood, or simply provide food for bacteria in the gut, which consequently multiply prolifically. Often, taking a supplement of digestive enzymes reduces the symptoms associated with food allergy and intolerance. Zinc supplementation can also be helpful, as deficiency of this mineral is extremely common among allergy sufferers. Zinc is not only needed for protein digestion, it's also essential for the production of hydrochloric acid in the stomach.

Cross-reactions

Another contributor to food sensitivity is exposure to inhalants that provoke a reaction. For example, it is well known that when the pollen count is high more people suffer from hay fever in polluted areas than in rural areas, despite lower pollen counts in cities. It is thought that exposure to exhaust fumes makes a pollen-allergic person more sensitive. Whether this is simply because their immune system or lungs have been weakened as a result of dealing with the pollution and are therefore less able to protect themselves from the additional pollen insult, or because some kind of 'cross-reaction' has taken place, is not known. In the USA, where sensitivity to ragweed is common, a cross-reaction with bananas has been reported. In other words, one sensitivity sensitises you to another. A similar cross-reaction may occur with pollen, wheat and milk for hay fever sufferers.

The emerging view, shared by an increasing number of allergy specialists, is that food sensitivity is a phenomenon caused by a number of factors, possibly including poor nutrition, pollution, digestive problems and over-exposure to certain foods. Removing the foods in question may help the immune system to recover, but other factors need to be dealt with as well if any major impact is to be made on long-term food intolerance.

Food Addicts

One interesting finding among people with food intolerances is that they often become hooked on the very food that causes a reaction, which can lead to bingeing on the foods that harm them most. Many patients describe the relevant foods as leaving them feeling drugged or dopey. In some cases the foods induce a mild state of euphoria. In this way, the food can act as a psychological escape mechanism from uncomfortable situations. But why do some foods cause drug-like reactions?

When pain, which alerts us to a physical problem no longer serves the body's needs, chemicals called endorphins are released. These are the body's natural painkillers: they make you feel better. The way they do this is by binding to sites on cells that turn off pain and turn on pleasant sensations. Opiates, such as morphine, are similar in chemical structure and bind to the same sites, which is how they suppress pain.

These endorphins, whether made by the body or taken as a drug, are peptides. Peptides are small groups of amino acids bound together – smaller than a protein and larger than a single amino acid. When the protein that you eat is digested, it first becomes peptides and then, if your digestion works well, single amino acids. In the laboratory, endorphin-like peptides have been made from wheat, milk, barley and corn (maize) using human digestive enzymes. These peptides have been shown to bind to endorphin receptor sites. Preliminary research does seem to show that certain foods, most commonly wheat and milk, may induce a short-term positive feeling, even if in the long term they are causing health problems.

Too often, the foods that don't suit you are the foods you feel you 'couldn't live without'. This is exactly what happens in the case of many food allergies. If you stop eating the suspect food you may get worse for a few days before you get better. Some things are addictive in their own right. These include sugar, alcohol, coffee, chocolate and tea (especially Earl Grey, which contains bergamot). You can react to these foods without being allergic. Wheat, corn and milk could be added to this list on the basis of their endorphin-like effects.

Reducing Your Allergic Potential

There are a number of possible reasons why a person becomes food-allergic. Among these are lack of digestive enzymes, leaky gut, frequent exposure to foods containing irritant chemicals, immune deficiency leading to hyper-sensitivity of the immune system, micro-organism imbalance in the gut lead-ing to leaky gut syndrome, and no doubt many more. Fortunately tests exist to identify deficiencies in digestive enzymes, leaky gut syndrome, and the balance of bacteria and yeast in the gut. These tests are not available on the NHS, but can be done through nutritionists and nutritionally-orientated doctors.

As well as identifying and avoiding foods that cause a reaction, there is a lot you can do to reduce your allergic potential.

Digestive enzyme complexes that help digest fat, protein and carbohy-drate (containing lipase for fat, amylase for carbohydrate and protease for protein) are well worth trying. Since stomach acid and protein-digesting enzymes rely on zinc and vitamin B6, it is worth taking 15mg of zinc and 50mg of B6 twice a day, as well as a digestive enzyme with each meal.

Leaky guts can heal. Cell membranes are made out of fat-like com-pounds, and one fatty acid, called butyric acid, helps to heal the gut wall. The ideal daily dose is 1200mg. The essential fatty acids – linoleic and linoenic acid – are also important for maintaining the right degree of gut permeability. Seeds such as sesame, sunflower and pumpkin contain good quantities of these substances. The vitamin biotin, together with B6, zinc and magnesium, helps the body to use these fatty acids properly. Vitamin A is also crucial for the health of any mucous membrane, including the gut wall. Supplementing these nutrients helps to heal a leaky gut.

Beneficial bacteria such as *Lactobacillus acidophilus* or *bifidus* can also help to calm down a digestive tract if the reaction is the result of a proliferation of the wrong kind of bacteria. If candidiasis is suspected, a more complex strategy is needed, and best carried out under the guidance of a nutrition consultant.

Immune boosting helps to reduce hypersensitivity of the immune system.

How to Test for Allergies and Intolerances

Of all the methods available for allergy testing, the only one I trust is the elimination diet. If avoidance of a particular food leads to reduction in symptoms, and reintroduction leads to worsening of symptoms, you know you have an intolerance to that food. It's worth checking the results of other tests you may have had carried out: avoid suspect foods and see if this makes a difference. The proof is in the eating, or rather, not eating.

Given that some foods may make you feel better in the short term and that some foods have a delayed reaction, it is best to avoid all suspect foods for at least fourteen and preferably thirty days. If you don't know what you're reacting to, you may get the best results by eating a very simple diet consisting of only foods with a low allergenic potential. The traditional elimination diet is lamb and pears. I prefer millet flakes, apple juice and an apple for breakfast, with quinoa or rice plus vegetables for lunch and dinner. These diets are hard to follow for more than fourteen days, as well as not being ideal nutritionally.

1. Completely avoid the suspect food for fourteen days.
2. On day 15 take your pulse at rest for sixty seconds.
3. Then eat more than usual of the food, e.g. three pieces of toast if you're avoiding wheat.
4. Take your pulse after ten, thirty and sixty minutes.

If your pulse goes up by 10 points, or if you have any noticeable symptoms within forty-eight hours, you probably have an allergy or intolerance to this food. The symptoms are more significant than the increased pulse, since some foods can raise your pulse without denoting an allergic reaction. If you are testing more than one food, and if the first food caused a reaction, wait

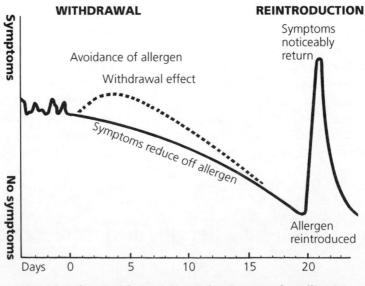

Fig. 14   The avoidance/reintroduction test for allergies

forty-eight hours before testing the next item. Otherwise reintroduce food number 2 the next day.

If you've ever had severe allergic reactions, and/or an attack of asthma, this test should not be carried out without the supervision of a doctor or nutritionist. If you suspect you have food allergies or intolerances, you would be well advised to see an ION-trained nutritionist who can help you identify what you are reacting to and advise on reducing your allergic potential.

Testing for IgG Allergies

The first type of tests to move away from measuring immediate IgE reactions were the 'cytotoxic' (toxic to cells) tests. These tests observe changes to the immune cells called neutrophils which clean up immune complexes caused by antibody–antigen reactions. Cytotoxic tests are thought to reflect IgG sensitivity.

The state-of-the-art method for measuring IgG sensitivity is a relatively new technique, developed during the 1990s, involving a method known as ELISA. It claims more reproducible and reliable results than cytotoxic testing, and indeed samples tested by both methods rarely agree in their results. One possibility is that these tests measure different types of reactions. Another is that one or both types of test is unreliable.

How Long to Avoid?

Just how long allergens have to be avoided is another open-ended question. Foods that invoke an IgE-type, immediate and pronounced reaction may need to be avoided for life. The 'memory' of IgE antibodies is long-term. In contrast, B-cells that produce IgG antibodies have a half-life of six weeks – which means that there are only half as many six weeks later. The 'memory' of these antibodies is therefore short-term, and within six months there is not likely to be any residual 'memory' of reaction to a food that's been avoided. While a six-month avoidance period may be ideal, Hoy and Braly report good results after as little as a month. Another option, after a strict one-month avoidance period, is to 'rotate' foods so that an IgG-sensitive food is only eaten every four days. This reduces the build-up of allergen–antibody complexes and reduces the risk of intolerance symptoms. Foods such as wheat and milk which are, by their nature, difficult to digest, are probably best avoided as much as possible.

TWENTY-ONE

THE GREAT BRITISH SPERM DISASTER

Something is going seriously wrong in human development. That's the conclusion of top-level scientists who have been monitoring crashing sperm counts and epidemic increases in hormonal, neurological and immune diseases over the past forty years. The threat of a drastic decline in fertility has brought this alarming trend to a head.

It's not, however, just fertility that's the concern. Linked in with this phenomenon is a higher incidence of certain cancers, most notably of the breast, cervix, testes and prostate gland, as well as a massive increase in allergies, asthma, eczema, rhinitis and migraines, now suffered by half of all children and adults. In addition, significant and ever-increasing developmental abnormalities point to factors capable of disturbing human development: undescended testes in boys, the development of enlarged breasts in older men, and the increased incidence of endometriosis, ovarian cysts and fibroids in women. To date, the scientific evidence points a finger at three main factors: pesticides, plastics and poor diet.

Pesticides – the Organochlorine Dilemma

Introduced in the 1930s to help reduce crop losses, chemical pesticides were heralded as a major boost to economic food production. There was, however, a sting in the tail, which didn't really get noticed until the 1960s.

The first family of pesticides were organochlorine compounds (OCs) such as DDT, dieldrin, Lindane and others. While highly effective as pesticides, they also proved highly toxic to man and very non-biodegradable; they are often present in the food chain twenty years after use. Most were banned in the USA in 1971 and voluntarily banned in the UK by 1979 (except for Lindane, which even today is permitted for some uses). Other OC compounds are still very much used in industry, while others continue to be sold illegally.

Despite the ban, levels in food and in humans remained relatively static. In 1987, for example, an analysis of baby foods found that 18 out of 31 samples had levels of dieldrin above EC Maximum Residue Levels (MRLs). Both Lindane and dieldrin are known to be carcinogenic and to reduce fertility. These OCs also have an oestrogenic effect (that is, they mimic the actions of oestrogen), which contributes to an overload of female hormones in men.

Organophosphates – out of the frying pan into the fire

With little market left for OCs, along came organophosphates (OPs), which now make up the largest class of pesticides, with over a hundred types on the market. Per annum we spend in the UK over £400 million on these chemicals. That's equivalent to 23.5 tonnes, or 420g per person. OPs' one advantage is that they are more biodegradable than OCs.

However, like OCs, many OPs are known to be carcinogenic, mutagenic (causing abnormal changes in cells) and toxic to the brain and nervous system. Forty per cent of pesticides now in use have been proved to be linked to cancer, birth defects or decreased fertility. OPs interfere with a vital brain neurotransmitter called acetylcholine: this messes up nerve transmission, which leads to loss of muscle coordination, convulsions and, when exposure is acute, death. Although deaths are rare (they are usually due to direct exposure in agricultural accidents), chronic exposure over long periods of time is not. Symptoms associated with long-term, low-level exposure include headaches, dizziness, insomnia, weakness, sweating, nausea, loss of appetite, disturbances in menstruation and infertility.

Despite these disturbing side-effects, OPs are in everything, from apples, carrots and lettuce even to your morning bowl of cornflakes. They are used to 'protect' grains while they're growing, and after harvesting to prevent weevil infestation. These foods are frequently found, on analysis, to contain OP residues above the safety levels set by the Ministry of Agriculture.

Widespread pesticide poisoning

While there are few provable cases of pesticide poisoning from normal food consumption, the circumstantial evidence for long-term effects is strong.

One neurological disease now closely linked to OPs is Parkinson's, the incidence of which is significantly higher among people who live in rural areas or other places where OPs are used. In Denmark, a comparison of organic farmers who consumed at least 50 per cent organic milk showed a significantly higher sperm count than in other milk drinkers. In the USA, researchers found a four-fold increase in soft-tissue cancer, and a doubling of the incidence of leukaemia, in children whose families' gardens had been treated with herbicides, pesticides or insecticides.

Harder to pin down is the relationship of OPs to the growing number of people who are allergic to chemicals and food. One study of 3300 people showed that 43 per cent had at lest one allergic symptom,[114] while in another study, of Swedish medical students, 46 per cent reported current or past allergies.[115] In a study undertaken in the USA by Professor William Rea, 99 per cent of 200 chemically sensitive patients were found to have, on average, three pesticides at levels above 0.05 parts per billion.[116] While we don't know the minimum level that causes problems, many such chemicals do cause a problem in the one part per billion range. The sum total of a number of chemicals could easily provide this kind of level and may well be a problem, particularly in sensitive people. Many allergic and chemically sensitive people also improve dramatically after changing to drinking spring or properly filtered water instead of tap water. In 1993, Professor Rea reported that the condition of 98 per cent of environmentally ill patients became better just by eliminating tap water. Approximately a quarter of all British tap water contains pesticides at levels above Maximum Admissible Concentrations. Professor Rea believes that symptoms like asthma, eczema, migraine, irritable bowl and rhinitis may be linked to pesticide exposure.

Dr Davies, a psychiatrist in rural Devon, where farming is a major industry, is convinced that pesticide exposure is also linked to depression, memory decline, schizophrenic reactions and destabilisation of moods, including outbursts of uncharacteristic aggression. Evidence also exists of a link between increased suicide rates and areas of the country where there is high OP use.

There is little scientific doubt that the current level of use of OP pesticides is contributing to a rapid decline in health and fertility. The Ministry of Agriculture is starting to encourage a switch to more organic farming methods. However, no serious steps have yet been taken to help bridge the price gap that exists between chemical-laden and organic food. A tax on pesticides, with the proceeds used to subsidise organic farming, for example, would be a feasible way for the government to put money where our mouths are.

Problems with Plastic

As discussed more fully in Chapter 9, a number of commonly occurring substances in plastics are now known to disrupt hormones and fertility. These include nonylphenols which can leach out of plastic products into foods, especially fatty ones. More insidious is their use in products such as spermicides in condoms and gels used with diaphragms. Nonylphenols – labelled as 'surfactants' – are found in dishwashing detergents and toiletries and are used as pesticides. Every year 18,000 tons are produced in the UK, and some ends up in our water supply. This is what is thought to be responsible for the infertility and feminising of fish in polluted rivers.

Based on the evidence to date, it would seem prudent to limit exposure of foods, particularly fatty ones, to plastic. But this is not always easy. Plastic packaging is used for most foods. Fatty snacks like crisps, or foods containing fat (e.g. cheese), wrapped in cling film are on the suspect list. Plastic in food packaging isn't always obvious, though. A layer of plastic lines cans and tetrapaks used for drinks. Those that aren't lined present another problem: they may leach dioxins (toxic agents used in bleaching paper and card). Dioxins are also used as pesticides and in industrial chemical processes. Although they are not oestrogen-mimickers, in a process that is not yet understood they have been shown in rodents to feminise males (physically and behaviourally) and are associated with infertility.

Environmental groups have been campaigning for legislation which would decrease our environmental load by banning nonylphenols and dioxins, but the list of commonly occurring hormone-disrupting chemicals is growing rapidly. What is perhaps of greatest concern is the finding that supposedly 'acceptable' levels of a number of chemicals produce a vastly exaggerated oestrogen effect when combined. As each new piece in the chemical jigsaw comes into view, the costs and the extent to which we need to clean up the environment, industrial processing and the food chain are growing.

Diet – the Missing Link

Nobody really suspects that modern diets aren't playing a part in this saga of chemical disease. The trouble is collecting evidence. Since the average diet contains foods laced with pesticides, is packaged in foods containing polychlorinated biphenyls (PCBs) and stored in plastic containing oestrogenic chemicals, it's very hard to prove what's doing what. So far, over four hundred toxic chemicals have been identified in human tissue analysis, and no doubt a similar number exist in the average diet. Once again, the particular worry is evidence of the combined effects of these toxins.

One could, of course, measure the health and fertility of those who eat highly packaged and chemically treated food against those who 'grow their own'. However, the diets would be so different that it would be impossible to identify the culprits.

Fat attack

What is known is that pesticides, PCBs and dioxins accumulate in fat. So one way to cut down your intake is to avoid high-fat foods, particularly of animal origin, since these chemicals exist throughout the food chain and accumulate so that they are in highest quantity at the top of the chain, among animals. Choosing skimmed milk rather than full-fat milk would decrease your load – even better if the milk is organic and in a glass bottle.

Fish concerns

Of course, you might think that if meat contains these chemicals fish would be better. But, unfortunately, due to the scale on which these chemicals have been used, most fish are now contaminated with PCBs and dioxins. Indeed, there is nowhere on this planet that isn't. Once again, they accumulate these toxins in fatty tissue, which, as for animals, is part of a defence mechanism against toxic compounds that are hard to eliminate. So whether fish is better or worse than organic meat is hard to say.

The fibre factor

Oestrogen is not an alien substance to the body, so it has in-built pathways for getting rid of excess. The main one is in bile, which is excreted into the digestive tract. Provided your diet contains enough fibre, your body can help to unload extra oestrogen-like chemicals through this channel.

Detox Nutrients

One factor that is probably highly underestimated is the role of micronutrients – vitamins, minerals and essential fatty acids – in protecting the body from these toxins. If you put a healthy man on a low-zinc diet, one of the earliest signs of deficiency is a drop in sperm count. Increase the zinc intake and sperm count returns to normal. Zinc, magnesium and molybdenum, for example, are needed to detoxify OPs. Many others are needed by the liver to transform fat-based toxins into substances that can be eliminated via the kidneys. This process, described more fully in Chapter 17, involves, among other nutrients, antioxidants such as vitamin A, C and E, zinc and selenium, plus a number of amino acids.

The integrity of body tissue and the digestive tract also acts, in part, as protection. Shortfalls in nutrients and essential fatty acids, which are used as building materials for these membranes, could increase risk of exposure. It is highly likely that a junk food diet, high in fried foods and low in micronutrients, may increase not only intake of toxic chemicals but also their absorption, and reduce the body's ability to eliminate them. General optimum nutrition guidelines must form a major part of any strategy for minimising the effects of unavoidable toxins and improving hormonal balance and fertility.

PART 6

FOOD FOR THOUGHT

The definition of insanity is to keep doing the same things and expect different results.

RITA MAY BROWN

TWENTY-TWO

CRIME – NOURISHMENT OR PUNISHMENT?

Almost everyone is a victim of crime at some time in their lives. During the 1990s we have witnessed a rapid increase in criminal behaviour, especially among young offenders. With fifty thousand people now in custody in the UK, at a cost of £500 per person per week, society has to question whether a criminal justice system based principally on punishment is the best solution and whether it is affordable.

Yet the fundamental question remains: how should a person who has committed a crime be treated? Punished as a deterrent? Removed from society to prevent further crime? Or should we be trying to understand the causes of deviant behaviour in order to rehabilitate the offender into society? In current rehabilitation practice, one factor that is completely overlooked is nutrition. Bernard Gesch, a former probation officer and now director of Natural Justice, a charity based in Cumbria, believes that the criminal justice system falsely places all the emphasis on social issues, ignoring physical factors such as nutrition. 'There are many chemicals around us that are known to affect behaviour. Our environment is increasingly polluted. Our food supply has fundamentally changed. In the same way that we don't notice ageing, how would we notice the effects of gradual changes to our diet and environment?' he asks. Yet the effects are clearly there.

The fact is that all thoughts, and consequently all behaviour, are processed through the brain and nervous system, which is totally dependent on the food we eat. Approximately half of all the glucose in the blood goes to power the brain, which is also dependent on a second-by-second supply of micronutrients – vitamins, minerals and essential fatty acids. Antinutrients such as lead and cadmium fundamentally affect brain function. 'What we're trying to do,' says Gesch, 'is introduce something new into the criminal justice system, that is the existence of the human brain.'

Sugar Blues

In a remarkable pilot project known as SCASO (South Cumbria Alternative Sentencing Options) young offenders were required, as part of their sentence, to undergo 'nutritional rehabilitation'. The participants were assessed for vitamin and mineral levels, toxic minerals and blood sugar balance, as well as general dietary intake. 'The most common problems were glucose intolerance and zinc deficiency. Every single person we tested had abnormal glucose tolerance on a five-hour glucose tolerance test,' says Gesch.[117] The importance of glucose control in relation to behaviour is a consistent finding among criminals. In Finland, a large number of habitual offenders were investigated for glucose balance.[118] Every single one had reactive hypoglycaemia (see below). In the USA, Professor Stephen Schoenthaler, head of the Department of Sociology and Criminal Justice at California State University, reported a 21 per cent reduction in anti-social behaviour, a 25 per cent reduction in assaults, a 75 per cent reduction in the use of restraints, and a 100 per cent reduction in suicides when 3000 inmates were placed on an experimental diet which reduced refined and sugary foods.[119]

Reactive hypoglycaemia is the term used to describe the rebound 'low' after a rapid increase in blood sugar levels induced by sugar, sweets or stimulants. It is associated with extreme tiredness, depression, aggression and attempted suicide. In other words, if you feel bad you're much more likely to behave badly. 'Of the forty to fifty people we worked with on SCASO we could create an impact in most in a week or two,' Gesch explained. Today's youth are like jet fighters. They refuel on the move, living off junk food, sweets and canned drinks.' His team taught the young offenders how to prepare simple and nutritious meals and to develop an interest in food.

Brain Pollution

One of the most invisible effects on behaviour is that of pollution. A worldwide consensus of research has shown that high lead levels equate to low intellectual performance and anti-social behaviour. The level of lead in the blood required to produce this effect is that commonly found in children in inner cities. One can therefore conclude that any child brought up in a polluted, inner city environment is affected to some extent. But you can't see the damage. The level of neurotoxins like lead that is needed to produce an effect on behaviour is just 1 per cent of that which produces physical symptoms. This is how sensitive the human brain is to environmental and nutritional changes.

Researcher Alex Schauss found significantly higher lead, cadmium and copper levels in violent, anti-social adults than in non-offenders.[120] Supplementing zinc, which is an antagonist of these heavy metals, had a favourable effect on behaviour. Neurotoxins such as lead and cadmium (of which cigarette smoke is a principal source) are largely unavoidable insidious brain pollutants.

Nutrients Against Crime

Nutritional deficiency is rife among young offenders, and Professor Schoenthaler found evidence of widespread folic acid, thiamine (vitamin B1) and vitamin C deficiencies. Just adding to their diets orange juice, which contains each of these nutrients, produced a staggering 47 per cent reduction in anti-social behaviour among juvenile offenders.[121] Deficiencies in calcium, magnesium, zinc, selenium and essential fatty acids have also been shown to correlate with increases in violent behaviour. Research by Schoenthaler in US prison populations showed that the simple addition of a multivitamin and mineral supplement containing RDA levels of nutrients has extremely positive effects on behaviour.

Anti-social Foods

Adverse reactions to foods are proving to be the fourth significant factor affecting behaviour. Severe allergic reactions can produce Jekyll and Hyde changes, as has been well reported in hyperactive children with chemical or food intolerances.[122] Although much harder to identify (and eliminate), the 3500 new chemicals that have been introduced into the food supply, as well as the over-consumption of wheat and milk (Britain's top two allergens), could be contributing to deviant behaviour, as illustrated by this case report from Dr Alex Schauss.

A president of a large American company, with no previous criminal record, goes for a drink at his local bar. For some reason he decides to have a glass of red wine, a drink he's never had before. Ten minutes later he pulls out a revolver and guns down a man walking past him. He shoots anyone who tries to help this man and ends up injuring twenty-two people. Miraculously, no one is killed, but many have serious wounds to their thighs, arms and upper bodies. A few hours later, in the local police station, he asks for a psychiatrist. When the psychiatrist arrives, the man asks: 'Why am I here?'

Fortunately this man was able to afford the best psychiatrist, neurologists and doctors, but none of them could find out what had triggered this atrocious action. The man himself could not even remember committing the crime, and was deeply horrified when he learned that he had done so. Tests eventually showed that he had a very imbalanced immune system and the common allergic symptoms of rhinitis and headaches.

The man was then tested for two months for sensitivity to various substances, including red wine – the likely offender. But, without any of the medical team's knowledge, he was simply being given placebos – non-reactive 'dummy' substances. Then, again without their knowledge, he was given exactly the same wine that he had drunk that fateful evening. Within ten minutes he became violent and aggressive, grabbing a nurse and tearing the laboratory apart. He was going through a Jekyll and Hyde-like metamorphosis: the psychiatrists present classified him as an acutely paranoid schizophrenic.

Twelve years before this incident, the man had moved to a very expensive block of flats in which a type of natural gas was used for heating and cooking. Sooner or later most people left their apartment because of the health-damaging effects of the gas, even though they had no chance of getting their money back. Pet birds had been known to die because of exposure to the gas. This man had spent seven years in the flat; it is likely that the gas considerably weakened his immune system, contributing to his aggressive reaction, which was probably to an 'amine' (a protein-like chemical) in the wine.

Who's to Blame?

The crux of the issue in criminal justice is culpability. If behaviour is thought of as purely a psychological/social phenomenon then the blame rests on individuals and their relationship with society. This kind of thinking results in our current strategy of punishment: removal from society and social rehabilitation. But if brain function and all the factors that affect it are put into the equation, the issues of nutrition and environmental pollution must be considered. The evidence of biochemical/nutritional imbalances presented in the SCASO case was so convincing that these factors were considered to be mitigating circumstances by the courts, resulting in less punitive sentences. These are, however, only isolated cases of individuals lucky enough to take part in pilot projects.

Diet vs Delinquency

The few studies conducted so far all show dramatic reductions in reoffending among individuals maintained on low-sugar, high-nutrient diets. According to Gesch, '75 per cent of our referrals were for violent offences, many of whom were multiple offenders. Of those kept on the combined social and nutritional regime none re-offended with a violent offence by the end of the six-month pilot study.'[123] The treatment provided (food supplements) cost between £4 and £10 a month. Compare that with the average cost of £2000 a month to keep someone in prison.

The first double-blind trial on young adults in a UK prison is under way, testing the effects of a multinutrient containing vitamins, minerals and essential fatty acids. Positive results, similar to those shown in US prison studies, may introduce a whole new element into the understanding of criminal behaviour.

TWENTY-THREE

ALZHEIMER'S – IS THERE AN ANSWER?

Trouble started at work. Just little things: she'd misfile a project, or forget the name of someone in the office. Then she forgot the way to the cafeteria. Her supervisor suggested that perhaps it was time she took retirement. Things started to go downhill from there. Her doctor dismissed her complaints as symptoms of the normal ageing process. It wasn't until Joan took a walk one winter afternoon, wearing her best summer dress on a snowy day, that her family finally believed something was seriously wrong.

This case, from neurologist Dr Jay Lombard and nutritionist Carl Germano, authors of *Brain Wellness Plan*, is typical. What could be worse than losing your mind, while your body still has many years to run? Yet that is precisely what happens to one in 10 people over the age of sixty-five, and one in 2 people over the age of eighty-five. With an ever-ageing population, Alzheimer's disease, the main cause of dementia, is being called 'the disease of the century'. The anxiety it brings, both to the sufferer and to their family, is immense. For many people on the slippery road to Alzheimer's, the first signs are depression, irritability, confusion and forgetfulness. Rather than wait until it's too late, now is the time to kick in with preventative measures.

According to psychiatrist Dr Abram Hoffer, Alzheimer's is a long time coming. He believes it is, like so many degenerative diseases, the long-term consequence of faulty nutrition and exposure to brain pollutants. Like so many diseases, many factors contribute to its initiation. These include:

- a genetic predisposition
- poor nutrition and digestive problems
- circulation problems
- viral infections
- toxic accumulation in the brain
- oxidant damage
- inflammation

Each of these can be prevented, with the exception of the genetic predisposition. The gene in question is called apolipoprotein E, or ApoE for short. It helps transport cholesterol and build healthy membranes for the brain's neurons. Those who inherit a particular type of this gene, called ApoE4, have three times the risk of developing Alzheimer's. The presence of this defective gene is now being used as a marker to predict risk.

Yet this risk may never become reality unless other circumstances prevail. One of these is infection with the herpes simplex virus, according to research carried out at Manchester's Molecular Neurobiology Laboratory and reported in the *Lancet* in 1997.[124] Indeed, recent research indicates that viruses can damages genes and the way in which they express themselves. Both vitamin E and selenium have been shown to stop viruses having this effect;[125] so it may be that only those deficient in these nutrients who are infected with the herpes virus increase their susceptibility to Alzheimer's. Vitamin E not only plays a key role in early prevention, but also in slowing down the progression of the disease. In a recent study reported in the *New England Journal of Medicine*, 341 Alzheimer's patients received either 2000ius of vitamin E or a placebo. Vitamin E was shown to reduce progression most significantly, thus relieving some burden on both patients and their families.[126] Dr Leon Thal of the University of California believes, 'The results of this study will be used to change the prescribing practices in the United States and probably many other parts of the world.'

Cardiovascular disease is another factor that increases the risk of Alzheimer's. A connection between the presence of ApoE4, atherosclerosis and increased Alzheimer's risk was made by Professor Hoffman at the Erasmus University Medical School in Rotterdam.[127] The most convincing theory is that blockages in arteries may lead to a poor supply of key nutrients to the brain. Without a good supply of antioxidants, for example, brain cells become more vulnerable to free radical damage.

Is Alzheimer's an Inflammatory Disease?

Another possibility is that both cardiovascular and Alzheimer's diseases may result from the same disease process. The diagnostic proof of Alzheimer's is the presence of plaques, or patches of dead cells and other waste material, in the brain. At the core of these plaques has been found a substance called beta-amyloid, an abnormal protein that is also found in the plaques of arterial deposits. Beta-amyloid is a toxic invader that results from the body being in 'emergency mode', resulting in inflammation as the immune system becomes over-reactive. It's a typical scenario that develops once a person's Total Environmental Load exceeds their capacity to adapt. Indeed, research has shown that taking anti-inflammatory drugs offers some protection from Alzheimer's, which is consistent with the hypothesis that the damage that occurs to brain cells is part of an overall inflammatory reaction. It also means that natural anti-inflammatory nutrients may prove to be important in prevention.

Inflammatory reactions invariably mean increased production of oxidants, hence an increased need for antioxidants such as vitamin A, betacarotene and vitamins C and E, all of which have been shown to be low in people with Alzheimer's. Also involved in calming down brain inflammation are essential fats. Particularly important is DHA, a type of omega-3 fat found in salmon, tuna, herring and mackerel. As well as being anti-inflammatory it is a vital component of brain cell membranes and helps control calcium flow in and out of cells. This factor is important because too much calcium inside brain cells is known to contribute to the production of the toxic beta-amyloid protein. DHA is available in fish oil supplements.

Another key membrane builder is a nutrient called phosphatidyl serine (PS), which also helps cells to communicate. Studies at the Vanderbilt University School of Medicine found that supplementation with PS improved memory, learning and other cognitive functions in Alzheimer's patients.[128]

Brain Pollution

Another brain toxin that is found in the plaques of Alzheimer's sufferers is aluminium. While plenty of studies have offered evidence of this increased accumulation of aluminium, what isn't clear is whether it is a cause or a consequence of the disease. Aluminium is known to accumulate with age, and in any event it's best to limit one's exposure to it. This means not cooking or storing food in aluminium pots, pans or foil, not using toothpaste packaged in aluminium tubes (plastic tubes are preferable, although may not be ideal, for reasons already discussed) and not taking antacids with added aluminium. To a certain extent zinc protects against aluminium and other metal toxicity, so a good zinc intake is another piece of the jigsaw.

Memory Boosters

Whatever the cause of the damage to brain cells the net consequence is lower levels of key neurotransmitters, which are produced within the brain's neurons. This slows down communication between cells and leads to memory loss and confusion. One of the key neurotransmitters is acetylcholine. Current research into Alzheimer's is focussing on ways to increase acetylcholine levels. Much like Prozac, which stops the breakdown of the neurotransmitter serotonin (deficiency of which is connected with depression), state-of-the-art Alzheimer's drugs block the breakdown of acetylcholine.

The alternative to these drugs is to supplement the nutrients the brain uses to make acetylcholine in the first place. These are choline and pantothenic acid (vitamin B5). Choline is most absorbable in the form of phosphatidyl choline. An alternative is DMAE, a substance that crosses readily into neurons and then converts into choline. The best dietary source of choline and DMAE is fish, especially sardines which are also rich in an important amino acid called pyroglutamate.

The discovery that the brain and cerebrospinal fluid contain large amounts of pyroglutamate led to its investigation as an essential brain nutrient. This amino acid is the building block of a whole new class of drugs called 'nootropics' (see Chapter 24), the best known of which is Piracetam. Studies using Piracetam have demonstrated clear improvement in memory, mood and cognitive abilities in both animals and humans.[129] One study, published in 1988 by Dr Pilch and colleagues, suggests that nootropics may increase the number of acetylcholine receptors in the brain.[130] Older mice were given Piracetam, a pyroglutamate derivative, for two weeks. Afterwards the researchers found that they had 30–40 per cent more acetylcholine receptors than before. This suggests that pyroglutamate-like molecules may also have a regenerative effect on the nervous system. The nutritional alternative is to supplement pyroglutamate itself.

The effects of enhancing mental performance through supplementation of 'smart nutrients' such as phosphatidyl choline, pantothenic acid, DMAE and pyroglutamate are likely to be far greater when taken in combination than individually. In a study in 1981, a team of researchers led by Raymond Bartus gave choline and Piracetam to aged lab rats – rats are noted from age-related memory decline.[131] The researchers found that, 'Rats given the Piracetam/choline combination exhibited [memory] retention scores several times better than those with Piracetam alone.' Their results also showed that half the dose was needed when Piracetam and choline were combined. Some 'brain food' supplements contain combinations of all these acetylcholine-friendly nutrients – choline, DMAE, pantothenic acid and pyroglutamate.

Oxygen – the Most Critical Nutrient

For any nutritional strategy to work, neurons must receive all the nutrients necessary for their normal function. None is more critical than oxygen. The transport of oxygen in the body is impaired by a deficiency of vitamin B12, folic acid, niacin or essential fats.

To keep cells running on oxygen requires much more than a good blood supply. Of the other nutrients that are essential to the use of oxygen in energy metabolism, the most important are vitamins B1 and B3, the anti-oxidant vitamins A, C and E, and the mineral selenium.

Vitamin B1 deficiency has long been known to result in brain damage. One of the most dangerous problems caused by excessive alcohol consumption is induced B1 deficiency, a condition called Wernicke–Korsakof Syndrome. The symptoms include anxiety and depression, obsessive thinking, confusion, defective memory (especially of recent events) and time distortion – not so different from Alzheimer's.

Vitamin B3 (niacin) is crucial for oxygen utilisation. It is incorporated into the co-enzyme NAD (nicotinamide adenosine dinucleotide), and many reactions involving oxygen need NAD. Without it, pellagra and senility can develop.

Optimum Nutrition – the Way Forward

But don't the elderly get enough of these vital vitamins? Sadly, the answer is an unequivocal 'no'. Anyway, enough is not always enough. Dr Abram Hoffer has shown that when cells have been starved of these nutrients they may become vitamin-dependent, requiring many hundred times the normal daily requirements.

One US study in 1975 examined the nutritional status of 93 geriatric patients and failed to find a single one with a normal nutritional profile.[132] The most common deficiencies were of vitamins C, E, A and B3. Other studies have frequently found elderly people to be deficient in folic acid, zinc, iron and calcium. To prevent the risk of heart and artery disease many researchers have recommended low-fat diets to older people and advised them to cut down on dairy produce and meat. Unfortunately this often leads to even worse iron, zinc and calcium status, unless proper dietary guidance and supplementation are given.

Alzheimer's disease may prove to be the consequence of decades of sub-optimal nutrition and exposure to neurotoxins from food and the environment. The ApoE4 gene may make some people more prone than others to mental deterioration, but this risk only becomes a reality under a certain set of circumstances. With optimum nutrition I believe that age-related memory impairment (suffered by 4 million people in Britain) and Alzheimer's can be prevented. As Leonard Larson, president of the American Medical Association in 1960, said, 'There are no diseases of the aged, but simply diseases among the aged.'

Nutrients to Prevent Alzheimer's

Nutrients	Prevention Dose	Intervention Dose
Vitamins and Minerals		
(found in multivitamin and mineral formulas)		
Vitamin A (Beta Carotene)	15,000ius	15,000–20,000ius
Thiamin (Vitamin B1)	50mg	250mg
Niacin (Vitamin B3)	100mg	500–1000mg
Pantothenic Acid (Vitamin B5)	100mg	300mg
Cyanocobalamin (Vitamin B12)	100mcg	1mg injection weekly
Vitamin C	2000mg	4000mg
Vitamin E	400ius	1000ius
Zinc	15mg	30mg
Selenium	200mcg	400mcg
Smart Nutrients		
(found in 'brain food' formulas)		
Phosphatidyl serine	100mg	300mg
Pyroglutamate	250mg	750mg
Choline	500mg	1000mg
DMAE	100mg	500mg
Other Nutrients		
Essential fat – DHA	150mg	300mg
Lipoic Acid	200mg	200mg
NAC (n-acetyl-cysteine)	500mg	1000mg
Gingko Biloba	150mg	300mg

TWENTY-FOUR

SMART DRUGS OR NUTRIENTS?

Your intelligence and memory aren't just genetically programed. Although there is clearly an in built element to intelligence, the development of learning skills and what you eat make a difference to your mental abilities.

The brain and nervous system, our mental 'hardware', are made up of a network of neurons, special cells which are each capable of forming tens of thousands of connections with others. Thinking is thought to represent a pattern of activity across this network. Such activity, or signals, involves neurotransmitters, the chemical messengers in the brain. When we learn, we actually change the wiring of the brain. When we think, we change the activity of neurotransmitters. Since both the brain and neurotransmitters are derived from nutrients in food, it is logical to believe that what you eat has a bearing on your mental performance.

In 1986 Gwillym Roberts, a schoolteacher and nutritionist from the Institute of Optimum Nutrition, and David Benton, a psychologist from Swansea University, decided to investigate whether an optimal intake of the nutrients used by the brain and nervous system would improve intellectual performance. Sixty schoolchildren were put on to either a special multivitamin and mineral supplement designed to ensure an optimal intake of key nutrients, or a placebo.[133] On analysing the diets of these schoolchildren before the trial it was discovered that a significant number were getting less than the RDA level of at least one nutrient. After eight months, the non-verbal IQs of those taking the supplements had risen by over 10 points! No changes were seen in those on the placebos, nor in a control group of children who had taken neither supplements nor placebos. (IQ tests have two sections: verbal and non-verbal. Verbal IQ is more influenced by schooling, while non-verbal IQ is considered more innate.)

Professor Stephen Schoenthaler, from the University of California, proposed that perhaps just a small percentage of schoolchildren whose IQs increased substantially were raising the average IQ difference in the whole sample group. Clearly supplements had an effect, but some questions were raised. Which children were benefiting from which supplements, and why? Which nutrients are important and at which levels? And how long does it take before any effect is noticed?

To answer some of these questions 615 schoolchildren in California were assigned to either a placebo group or one of three 'supplement' groups given approximately 50, 100 or 200 per cent of the US RDAs for vitamins and minerals.[134] After one month, only the 200 per cent RDA group had significantly higher IQ scores than the placebo group. After three months, all supplement groups had higher IQ scores than the placebo group, with the 100 per cent RDA group having the highest, and statistically most significant, increase. Of this group 45 per cent had an increase in IQ of 15 or more points, compared to the average increase of 4.4 points.

Following these initial studies, at least ten more have been performed. All bar two showed similar results – an increase in non-verbal IQ score in those taking vitamin and mineral supplements. So why did two studies fail to find this effect? The first, carried out by researchers from King's College, London, gave supplements to schoolchildren for only one month, compared to seven months in the original trial. It takes time, it seems, for improvement in mental performance to take effect. On examining the second study that showed negative results undertaken by Dr Crombie and colleagues testing children in Dundee, Scotland, Professor Schoenthaler found that the two groups (supplement and placebo) were not evenly matched. There were two children with very high IQs in the supplement group, who were introducing a bias into the results. Once these two children were taken out of the figures, this study, like the others, showed a consistent increase in non-verbal IQ amongst those taking supplements.

Why Do Vitamins Raise IQ?

But how does improved nutrition increase IQ scores? A recent study by Wendy Snowden from Reading University's Department of Psychology offers an explanation: once again, schoolchildren were given either supplements or placebos.[135] The supplemented children showed significant increases in non-verbal IQ scores (but not in verbal IQ scores) after ten weeks. A close analysis of performance in the IQ tests showed the same error rate in both groups but fewer questions left unanswered by the supplemented children. Since almost all the unanswered questions were towards the end of the test, when the children ran out of time, it would seem that those on supplements answered the questions faster (hence fewer unanswered). This suggests that the effect of the vitamin and mineral supplements was to increase the speed of processing, which is clearly a significant factor in IQ performance and presumably in intelligence.

In the verbal IQ test all the children completed all the questions, so there was no possibility of improvement in the numbers unanswered.

Memory Boosters

Although studies have yet to be performed to prove it, there is no good reason to assume that adults can't achieve similar benefits in sharpening their intelligence through optimum nutrition. But what about sharpening your memory? Chapter 23 looked at Alzheimer's disease, the ultimate in memory loss. But what about the milder and more commonly experienced memory decline that we tend to ascribe to the normal process of ageing or simply to personality differences? Is there room for improvement here?

According to the drug companies, there is. 'Age-associated memory impairment affects many more people than Alzheimer's disease, although, it's certainly true, it is a much less severe condition. We believe at least 4 million people in the UK suffer from this,' says Dr Paul Williams from Glaxo pharmaceuticals, who have been developing drugs to enhance memory and mental performance. A report in the *Economist* magazine (1993) says, 'The American pharmaceutical industry is developing more than 140 types of smart pills in its laboratories, making them the tenth-largest class of drugs being researched.' Even larger than the market for an Alzheimer's cure is the market for ways of dealing with the new 'disease' of Age-Associated Memory Decline (AAMI). Just as with 'attention deficit disorder', once it is recognised as a disease doctors will be able to prescribe smart drugs to those who consider their memory needs a boost. So what are these drugs, and do they work?

Smart Drugs

With a hundred 'smart drugs' already developed, this subject is material for a book in itself. (The best books currently available are *Smart Drugs and Nutrients* and *Smart Drugs 2 – The Next Generation* by Dr Ward Dean and John Morgenthaler.) Many of these drugs fall into one or other of two categories:

- Drugs which block the breakdown of neurotransmitters and so keep more of these substances in circulation
- Drugs which mimic the action of hormones or neurotransmitters

The neuro-immuno-endocrine network and the way neurotransmitters and hormones help us to keep adapting to our environment was discussed in Chapter 5. As we age, levels of these hormones and neurotransmitters tend to fall, and as a result our ability to maintain optimal mental and physical health declines.

Two of the most popular smart drugs are Deprenyl and Piracetam. Deprenyl, also called selegiline, is now used for the treatment of both Parkinson's and Alzheimer's disease. Some people recommend taking it to prevent these diseases as a general stimulant to mental functioning, even when no symptoms are present. In animals it has also been shown to extend lifespan. Chemically, it is part of a group of drugs called mono-amino-oxidase inhibitors, or MAOIs for short. These are also used as antidepressants. They work by stopping neurotransmitters from being broken down. Deprenyl has a better track record than a number of MAOI drugs, which have unpleasant side-effects. However, it is still a drug that interferes with the body's natural biochemistry.

Piracetam is one of a number of new drugs called nootropics, which are related to the amino acid pyroglutamate. Over 150 studies on Piracetam have been published; they show it to have a broad effect on enhancing mental performance. Numerous studies have shown improvements in memory, concentration, coordination and reaction time.[129] The drug is also being used with reasonable success in the treatment of Alzheimer's (see Chapter 23).

For the pharmaceutical industry, the advantage of these drugs is that they are not nutrients but man-made substances – in other words, they can be patented after vast sums have been spent on research. The disadvantage of such man-made chemicals is that, although modelled on nutrients, they are alien to the human body. They never produce a perfect fit in enzyme systems and, while creating the desired effect in the short term, can, in the long term, imbalance the body chemistry. Of course, the long-term effects of most of these new smart drugs have yet to be discovered.

Smart Hormones

One step closer to nature is the use of 'smart hormones' – naturally occurring hormones that have an effect on performance. In this category come melatonin, pregnenolone and DHEA. In the USA, these natural hormones are sold over the counter to deal with anything from jetlag to life extension. In the UK they are only available on prescription.

Although they occur naturally, these substances are not without side-effects. DHEA and pregnelonone can, if needed, be turned into oestrogen and testosterone. Pregnenolone can also be turned into progesterone. So they can have a powerful effect on the balance of the sex hormones, as well as on the adrenal hormones which are involved in the stress response.

Both DHEA and pregnenolonone levels tend to decrease with age, and the simplistic view is that supplementing them will stop you ageing. The trouble is, if you have more than you need the body has to work hard to get rid of the excess. Where these hormones are concerned, more is not necessarily better.

While potentially useful for those with adrenal exhaustion, blood sugar problems and hormonal imbalances, they are not recommended for supplementation except under the guidance of a practitioner. Before-and-after tests should be carried out to determine whether or not there is a deficiency, in which case correcting it is likely to improve mental functioning. The older you are, the more likely you are to have low levels of DHEA and pregnenolone. For this reason many older people on the USA supplement up to 25mg of DHEA a day. More than this is unwise without proper testing.

Melatonin became famous as the answer to jetlag. It is a hormone produced by the pineal gland, the master gland of the endocrine system, which conducts the orchestra of other hormone-producing glands that control blood sugar levels, stress reactions, sex hormones, calcium balance and other critical processes in the body.

The pineal gland also acts as a biological clock, secreting melatonin during the night. Long-distance travelling upsets this system and can result in the well-known jetlag symptoms – fatigue, fuzzy thinking, insomnia and headaches. After taking melatonin in the evening in the new time zone many people experience a substantial reduction in these symptoms.[136] More controversial is the recommendation to take melatonin for depression, for memory enhancement or for extending lifespan. Given at the wrong time of day it can worsen mental functioning, creating the equivalent of jetlag. Of all the smart hormones I recommend the most caution when using melatonin, except possibly for seasonal affective disorder (SAD) and short-term use in correcting jetlag. In these situations 5mg in the evening may be worth experimenting with, under the guidance of a health practitioner.

Smart Nutrients

There is an alternative and safer way to get your neuro-immuno-endocrine network zinging. That is to ensure that you are taking in through your diet optimal levels of the nutrients from which your body can make all these key neurotransmitters and hormones.

Acetylcholine, the memory neurotransmitter, is made from the nutrient choline, together with pantothenic acid (vitamin B5). Choline is abundant in fish, especially sardines. Pyroglutamate is found in many foods, including fish, fruit and vegetables. Optimal intakes of niacin (vitamin B3), folic acid and B12 all help to keep your neurotransmitters in circulation.

Another nutrient, phosphatidyl serine, has memory-enhancing properties. In a study by Dr Thomas Crook and colleagues 149 people with age-associated memory impairment were given a daily dose of 300mg of phosphatidyl serine or a placebo. When tested after twelve weeks, those taking the phosphatidyl serine showed improved memory and mental function.[137]

Essential fats, especially DHA which is found in fish, are particularly important for mental development during pregnancy and infancy. Glutamine, another amino acid that is a building block for neurotransmitters, can be used as fuel for the brain and has been shown to enhance mental performance and decrease addictive tendencies.[138]

These are worthy additions to a supplement programme designed to promote optimal mental performance and prevent age-related memory decline. Many can be found in combination in smart nutrient supplements. I recommend the following:

Guide to Smart Nutrients

*Niacin or niacinamide (B3)	150mg
*Pantothenic acid (B5)	300mg
Folic acid	400mcg
Vitamin B12	100mcg
*Phosphatidyl choline	1000mg
or DMAE	50g
*Pyroglutamate	450mg

*All these are available in one supplement called Brain Food,
  manufactured by Higher Nature (see Directory of Supplement Manufacturers)

If you are over fifty or suffering from age-related memory decline,
add the following:

Phosphatidyl serine	100mg
DHEA	25mg
Glutamine	5000mg

These nutrients are supplements to an optimal diet, which needs to include fish three times a week, preferably salmon, mackerel, tuna or herring. For vegetarians a good source of protein such as tofu is essential, as is a source of the essential fatty acid DHA, which can be made from linolenic acid (richest in flax seeds and pumpkin seeds, but also available derived from algae). You need a tablespoon of DHA a day.

PART 7

FOOD FOR THE FUTURE

Let food be your medicine and medicine be your food.

HIPPOCRATES

TWENTY-FIVE

SUPERFOODS

Imagine getting a prescription from your doctor for broccoli, garlic and wheatgrass. This is the scenario that scientists are predicting, as more and more phytochemicals are discovered. Phytochemicals are active compounds in food that prevent disease. Indoles, found in cabbage and Brussels sprouts, have anti-cancer properties. Chlorophyll, in green plants, helps to oxygenate the blood and improve energy. Allicin, in garlic and spring onions, boosts the immune system. These are just three of hundreds of the commonly occurring phytochemicals in nature's pharmacy.

Although many of these are not classified as essential nutrients (in other words, our lives do not depend on them), they do impact on the chemistry of the body and on our health as significantly as vitamins and minerals. Many foods contain a combination of these health-promoting phytochemicals and essential nutrients. Instead of using pharmaceutical drugs with undesirable side-effects, the medicine of tomorrow is turning to nutraceuticals to correct the body's chemistry and restore wellbeing. Every time you eat living foods, fruit and vegetables, you take in a cocktail of essential vitamins, minerals, amino acids, antioxidants, enzymes and phytochemicals that work together to promote your health. The idea of separating each ingredient and treating it like an individual drug to cure a specific illness is not only impractical but nonsensical.

Food as Medicine

With the discovery of more and more phytonutrients, medicine is coming full circle and starting once again to embrace the words of Hippocrates – let food be your medicine. Certain foods have been found to be particularly powerful health promoters. It is highly beneficial to include these 'superfoods' in your daily diet.

Aloe vera

Extracts of aloe vera first became popular as a skin healer. Aloe actually accelerates fibroblast development, which is necessary for collagen repair and wrinkle prevention. But recent research shows that this ancient remedy does much more. It is a powerful detoxifier, antiseptic and tonic for the nervous system. It also has immune-boosting and antiviral properties. Exactly what the active ingredient is remains a bit of a mystery. Aloe vera is rich in mucopolysaccharides, one of which is called acemannan, but also contains lignins, enzymes and antiseptic agents plus vitamins, minerals, essential fats and amino acids. Research by Dr Jeffrey Bland found that adding aloe vera to one's daily diet improved digestion, absorption and elimination.[139] As such, it is an aid to digestion.

There is some controversy about the best source. Most authorities agree that too much aloin, an ingredient in the outer flesh, has a purgative effect. So some aloe vera product companies fillet the leaf to produce a gel from the inner part. Others process the whole leaf in such a way as to remove the aloin. Concentration also varies from one product to another. Technicalities aside, there seems great advantage in taking a measure of aloe vera each day as a general health tonic.

Berries

All fruits with a purple/blue colour such as black grapes, bilberries, cranberries, blackcurrants and blueberries are especially rich in a type of flavonoid called anthocyanidins and proanthocyanidins. These phytonutrients are very powerful antioxidants and anti-inflammatory agents. They are substantially stronger than vitamin E in this regard[140] and are well worth including in your diet, either by eating berries when available or by supplementing concentrated extracts. Many advanced antioxidant formulas now contain a source of these flavonoids, for example bilberry extract.

Blue-green algae

These organisms are at the very bottom of the food chain and represent the purest nutrition you can get, being rich in chlorophyll, vitamins, minerals, essential fats and phytonutrients.

Spirulina is a blue-green alga which flourishes in the warm-water lakes of Mexico and Africa. It is 60 per cent protein and an excellent source of essential fats including GLA, as well as vitamins and minerals. It is especially rich in betacarotene – 3g of spirulina provide as much as 16,000ius. Spirulina has been shown to have numerous health benefits, particularly in relation to arthritis, immune system enhancement and skin problems. It is a worthwhile addition to a supplement programme at around 3g a day. Quality can vary – go for high-quality organic.

Chlorella, like spirulina, is rich in protein, vitamins, minerals and chlorophyll.

Klamath Lake Blue-Green Algae is a particular species (*Aphanizomenon flos-aquae*) which is only found in Klamath Lake in Oregon, USA. The lake is very nutrient-rich due to run-off from several rivers which originate in the surrounding mountains, and it is abundant in this alga which is harvested and freeze-dried. It has similar benefits to spirulina. As with all algae products, quality can vary – so choose carefully.

Carrots, sweet potatoes, watercress and peas

All these foods are very rich in carotenoids and betacarotene, as well as other nutrients. They're great to eat on a regular basis. Sweet potatoes can be baked, boiled or mashed and are great in soups. A carrot a day may indeed keep the doctor away.

Cruciferous vegetables

These members of the brassica family are rich sources of the anti-cancer phytochemicals called isothiocyanates. They include broccoli, Brussels sprouts, cabbage, cauliflower, cress, horseradish, kale, kohlrabi, mustard radish and turnip, and have been linked to a reduced risk of cancer. Research has shown that if you eat these foods every day you halve your cancer risk.[141] Both broccoli and Brussels sprouts are increasingly protective against cancer, the more you eat. One particular phytochemical in these foods, glucosinolate, has been shown to increase liver detoxification potential significantly[142] – a 30 per cent increase was achieved by eating three servings of Brussels sprouts a day.

Essential oils

In spite of the bad name given to fats, there are two we cannot live without. These are omega-3 and omega-6 fatty acids. From these two families of fats the body makes cell membranes, brain tissue and prostaglandins, powerful hormone-like substances that control cardiovascular health, fertility, sex hormones, brain and nerve function, skin health and a host of other essential processes.

Almost all food processing damages essential fats and they rapidly become rancid, so food manufacturers have carefully kept them out of modern food. Any kind of frying not only destroys these oils in food, but damages them so that they have a detrimental effect. The consequence is that our modern diet is devoid of fresh seeds and their oils, but abundant in processed and cooked food. This produces both fatty acid deficiency and an imbalance between these two important nutrients. In fact, approximately three-quarters of the population is grossly deficient in essential fats, while the average person today gets one-sixth of the intake of omega-3 oils that people did in the nineteenth century.

One of the simplest ways to prevent deficiency and correct the balance is to have one or two tablespoons of the right kind of oils every day, added to salads, soups, cereals and other food after cooking. Two such oil blends, which consist of combinations of organic sesame, sunflower and borage oil (rich in omega-6) and flax and pumpkin oil (rich in omega-3) are called Essential Balance™ and Udo's Choice. Both are available in light-proof containers from health food stores. A tablespoon a day ensures an optimal intake of essential fats.

Fish

Quite apart from being a good source of protein, vitamins and minerals (especially selenium), fish are also rich in many brain-enhancing nutrients including choline and DMAE. The fatty or carnivorous fish – salmon, tuna, shark, swordfish, mackerel and herring – are excellent sources of the essential fats DHA and EPA. These omega-3 fats are particularly associated with health improvements, including the reduction of risk for cardiovascular disease, balancing hormones and improving mental function. They are certainly essential during pregnancy and infancy for proper mental development. While these essential fats can be derived from alpha-linolenic acid, which is particularly concentrated in flax seeds, the body is poor at converting it. For this reason a direct source of DHA and EPA may be preferable. This means eating fish three times a week, or taking concentrated fish oil capsules. Look out for EPA/DHA advertised as PCB-free. For vegetarians there is now a concentrated source of DHA, extracted from a specific alga, available in capsules.

Garlic

For thousands of years people have been aware of the beneficial properties of garlic. The slaves who constructed the pyramids of Egypt were given garlic cloves daily to sustain their strength, as were Roman soldiers. Back in 1858 Louis Pasteur confirmed that garlic had antibacterial effects, and it was used to treat infection before the days of more specific antibiotics. Garlic contains around two hundred biologically active compounds, many of which play a role in preventing diseases. Principal among these compounds is a substance called allicin, which is antiviral, antifungal and antibacterial. Garlic also acts as an antioxidant, being rich in sulphur-containing amino acids.

Studies from China show that people who eat a lot of garlic are protected against stomach cancer.[143] This may be because garlic is able to block the conversion of nitrites and nitrates (found in many preserved foods) into cancer-causing nitrosamines. Garlic can also inhibit the action of aflatoxins, which are naturally occurring substances found in peanuts, that can cause cancer. The results of a large study involving 41,837 women aged between 55 and 69 from Iowa, USA, indicated that garlic was the most protective type of vegetable against colon cancer. Women who said they ate garlic at least once a week were 50 per cent less likely to contract colon cancer than those who said they never ate it.[144]

Garlic significantly lowers cholesterol in the blood and prevents the formation of atherosclerosis. A three-year study at Tagore Medical College in India divided over four hundred patients who had already suffered heart attacks into two groups. One group were given garlic supplements equal to six to ten cloves per day. They suffered fewer heart attacks and had significantly lower cholesterol counts than the group who did not take garlic.[145] Garlic also helps prevent blood clots – probably a safer way to maintain thin blood than taking an aspirin a day, which can cause stomach bleeding. According to medical trials, garlic also reduces the risk of heart attacks by significantly lowering cholesterol in the blood and preventing the formation of atherosclerosis.

There's no doubt that garlic is an important ally in fighting infections, and a wise inclusion in one's diet. Have a clove or capsule every day, and more if you're fighting an infection.

Power mushrooms

Two species of mushrooms, shiitake and reishi, possess immune-enhancing properties. Shiitake mushrooms are particularly popular in Japan and are now available in British supermarkets. You can also buy them dry and soak them before cooking. They are an extremely nutritous food and one of the few vegetable sources of vitamin D. Rich in calcium and phosphorus, they also contain high levels of many amino acids including leucine, lysine and threonine, plus the phytochemical lentinan, a powerful immune stimulant which appears to inhibit virus replication. In animal studies it has been shown to have anti-tumour properties. Lentinan is widely used to treat cancer in Japanese hospitals. It also induces the production of interferon, the body's own antiviral chemical used to fight off infection. Other research suggests that lentinan may have potential in the fight against AIDS. It has demonstrated anti-HIV activity and, in one US study, 30 per cent of patients taking lentinan who were HIV+ showed an increase in their T cell counts after twelve weeks, indicating improved immunity.[146]

Another immune-boosting mushroom is reishi, which has long been revered in the East for its healing powers. Although there are at least seven species with many different colours, the red *Ganoderma lucidum* is regarded as the king. As it's tough and indigestible in its natural form, it must be cooked or processed first in order to release the nutrients. Traditionally it is decocted as a tea or ground into a powder which can be added to soups and stews. It can also be taken as a capsule or liquid tincture. It is currently the most widely used medicinal mushroom for immune disorders in the East. The Chinese believe reishi is effective for treating a host of diseases including hepatitis, bronchitis, bronchial asthma, coronary disease, gastric ulcers, stomach ache and migraine. Recent medical research has demonstrated reishi's wide range of adaptogenic properties including blood sugar regulation, immune support, free radical protection effects, cholesterol-lowering properties, sedative and antihypertensive effects. Potent antiallergic activity has been reported, including antihistamine actions, and it is being used in Japan to help alleviate some of the toxic side-effects of radiotherapy and chemotherapy in cancer patients.

Quinoa

Pronounced 'keenwa', this is a staple food in the high Andes. Grown for five thousand years and reputed to be the source of strength of the Aztecs working in high altitudes, it is proving to be food for the gods. Known as the 'mother grain' for its unique sustaining properties, it contains significantly more protein than any grain, with a quality of protein better than meat. It's also rich in vitamins and minerals, providing almost four times as much calcium as wheat, plus extra iron, B vitamins and vitamin E. Not technically a grain but a seed, as such quinoa is rich in polyunsaturated oils, providing essential fatty acids. It is about as close to a perfect food as you can get, and can be found in many health food stores. Add two parts of water to one of quinoa and boil for fifteen minutes. It's good with vegetable and tofu steam-frys.

Seeds and nuts

Nuts and seeds are rich sources of essential fats, vitamin E and many minerals including calcium, magnesium, zinc and selenium. While nut and seed consumption has declined due to fat phobia, I recommend eating them every day and cutting down instead on sources of saturated animal fat (from meat and dairy produce) and hydrogenated vegetable oils (from processed foods). Healthy men placed on diets containing walnuts have shown a significant decrease in cholesterol levels after only four weeks compared to those following a similar diet with the same fat content but no nuts, according to research published in the *New England Journal of Medicine*. Other nuts such as almonds and hazelnuts have also been shown to have beneficial effects on cholesterol.

One of the richest known sources of omega-3 fats is flax seed. This small brown seed was revered by the Cherokee Indians, who believed that it captured energies from the sun that were vital to the body, increased virility, nourished a woman during pregnancy and healed skin diseases and arthritis. All these healing properties have since been proved by modern science. Pumpkin seed and hemp seed are also reasonable sources. Omega-6 fats are found in abundance in sesame and sunflower oil. To get a balance of both families of essential fats mix sesame, sunflower and flax seeds, keep them in a sealed jar in the fridge, and eat a heaped tablespoon every day.

Soya products and tofu

These are both excellent sources of protein and isoflavones, which are powerful phytoestrogens. Isoflavones are known to decrease the risk of hormone-related cancers including those of the breast and prostate gland. Two particular isoflavones have been identified: genistein and diadzein. An ideal intake for cancer prevention is around 100–200mg a day. This is equivalent to a 350ml (12fl.oz) serving of soya milk or a 75g (3oz) serving of tofu.

Watermelon

This fruit is a fine example of what wonderful benefits you can get from natural foods. The flesh is very rich in the antioxidants vitamin C, lycopene and carotenoids including betacarotene. The seeds are rich in vitamin E, essential fats, selenium and zinc. Put both flesh and seeds in a blender to make watermelon juice, a natural antioxidant cocktail ideal for fighting infections and pollution and for detoxifying diets.

Wheatgrass and barleygrass

Packed full of nutrients, 'green foods' such as these are among the richest natural source of antioxidants and chlorophyll. Chlorophyll is what makes plants green. It is highly cleansing, alkalising and full of minerals, especially magnesium. The nutrients contained in cereal grasses are more like those of a dark green vegetable than those of a grain, so they are gluten-free and safe for coeliacs (people allergic to gluten). There are hundreds of enzymes in cereal grasses; some of the most significant to be found in wheatgrass include the antioxidants cytochrome oxidase, required for proper cell respiration, and superoxide dismutase. Other enzymes such as lipase, protease and amylase are extremely beneficial for digestion.

The plants grow slowly throughout the winter, accumulating vitamins and minerals and storing them in their leaves. This grass stage lasts for about two hundred days, then, as the plants reach their nutritional peak in the spring, they begin to form a joint which will go on to produce the stalk of grain. Once jointing occurs the levels of nutrients drop dramatically, as they are now needed for the production of the grain. So the grass is usually harvested just before jointing, using only the top 7–8cm – the most nutritious part of the plant. The leaves can then be dried at a low temperature and turned into tablets or powders which can be added to drinks.

Future Foods

As the link between food and health, and the awareness of this link, grows stronger, food will be marketed and grown for its health-promoting properties. Special strains of plants will be sought out that increase their phytonutrient effect. Plants will also be grown in mineral enriched soil. Organic produce will become commonplace. There is every reason to suspect that the quality of food will improve, for those who choose it.

But remember this: however ingenious humans may be, our bodies have been shaped over millions of years, adapting to a natural environment. Pure, unadulterated food is what we've adapted to, what our bodies need – and that is not going to change. So make sure that most of your diet consists of whole, natural food that you could pull out of a tree, or pull from the ground, free from pesticides, artificial additives or genetic modifications. Chapter 26 explains what this means in terms of your daily diet.

TWENTY-SIX

DIET FOR THE NEW MILLENNIUM

Food is medicine. Some of it is good medicine, and some bad. Yet every single meal you eat is contributing to or taking away from your health and longevity. The question is this: do you eat to live, or live to eat? Most people select food on the basis of what makes them feel good in the short term by giving immediate taste satisfaction, without contemplating the idea that today's feast can be tomorrow's downfall.

As you become increasingly aware of the power of food in relation to health, the process of eating becomes two things: an act of pleasure and a boost to your health. Many of the healthiest foods taste great. That's why the best chefs go to great lengths to buy fresh, organic produce. It tastes better.

Throughout this book you've learned about different food factors that will help promote your health. For example, you've discovered that eating cabbage, broccoli and Brussels sprouts three times a week cuts your risk of colon cancer by 60 per cent; and that eating garlic every day almost halves your risk of stomach cancer. All these important findings are allowing us to define a diet for the new millenium – a way of eating that will go a long way to eradicating the diseases from which we now suffer and die, and maximise our chances for a long and healthy life.

In addition to following general guidelines for an optimal diet (shown overleaf) here are some specific recommendations and foods to include in your weekly menu, plus some examples of what this means on your plate:

Eat foods raw or lightly cooked

All cooking destroys nutrients, but slow cooking, steaming or simple short cooking methods (see below) minimise nutrient losses. (However for some very fibrous vegetables, such as leeks, cooking helps break down cell membranes which can actually make more nutrients available.) In general, try to eat most of your food raw or just lightly cooked.

Add colour to your diet

Natural colours in food are due to phytochemicals. Tomatoes and water-melon get their colour from the antioxidant lycopene. Carotenoids such as betacarotene make carrots, apricots, melons and mangoes orange. Mustard and turmeric are yellow thanks to curcumin, a natural anti-inflammatory agent. Green food is rich in chlorophyll and magnesium. The purple colour in blueberries, blackberries, red grapes and cherries is a rich source of the important anti-oxidants anthocyanidins and proanthocyanidins.

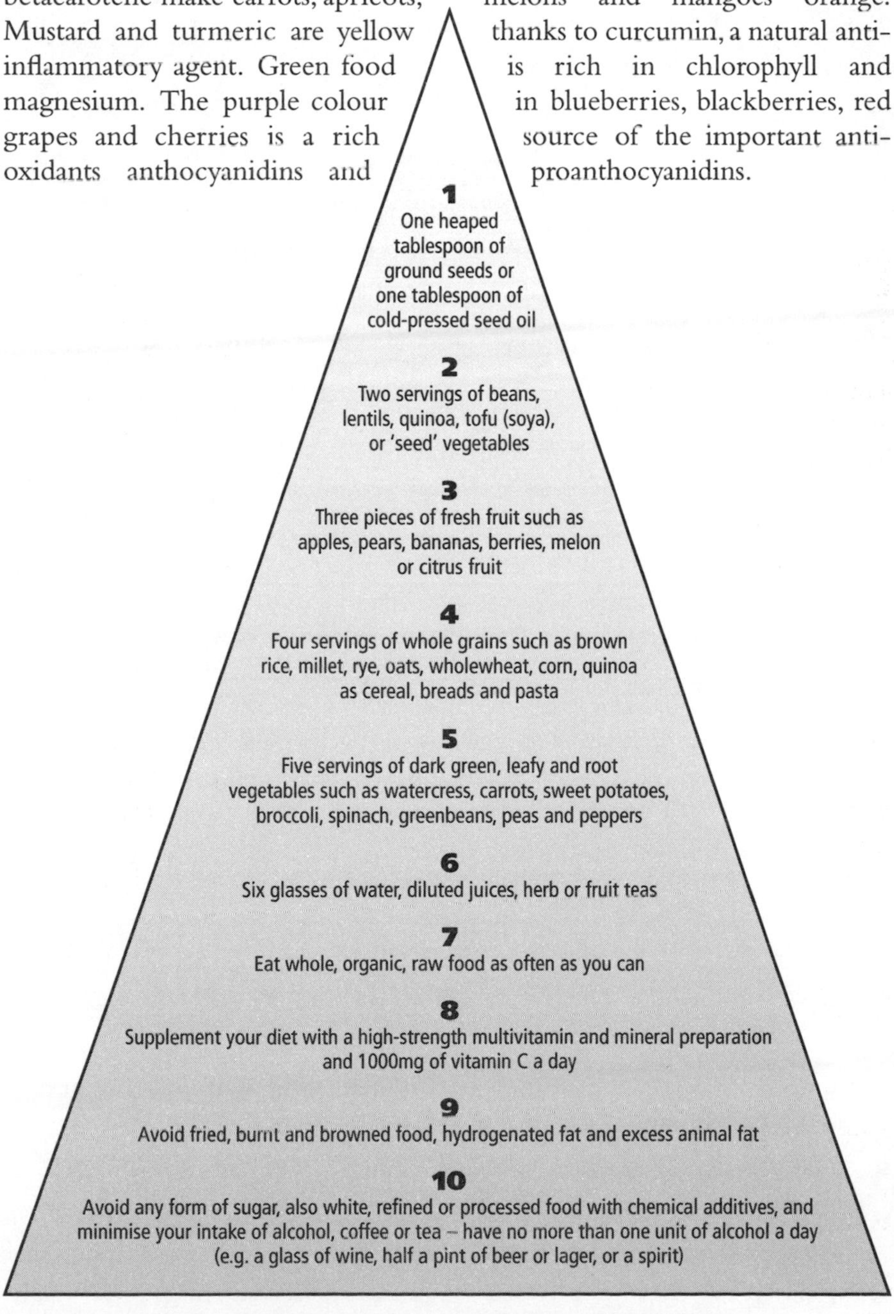

1
One heaped tablespoon of ground seeds or one tablespoon of cold-pressed seed oil

2
Two servings of beans, lentils, quinoa, tofu (soya), or 'seed' vegetables

3
Three pieces of fresh fruit such as apples, pears, bananas, berries, melon or citrus fruit

4
Four servings of whole grains such as brown rice, millet, rye, oats, wholewheat, corn, quinoa as cereal, breads and pasta

5
Five servings of dark green, leafy and root vegetables such as watercress, carrots, sweet potatoes, broccoli, spinach, greenbeans, peas and peppers

6
Six glasses of water, diluted juices, herb or fruit teas

7
Eat whole, organic, raw food as often as you can

8
Supplement your diet with a high-strength multivitamin and mineral preparation and 1000mg of vitamin C a day

9
Avoid fried, burnt and browned food, hydrogenated fat and excess animal fat

10
Avoid any form of sugar, also white, refined or processed food with chemical additives, and minimise your intake of alcohol, coffee or tea – have no more than one unit of alcohol a day (e.g. a glass of wine, half a pint of beer or lager, or a spirit)

Fig. 15   Top ten daily tips for an optimal diet

Choose natural, organic and whole foods

Select foods as close to their natural form as possible – organic if you can. On average it is 25 per cent more expensive, but it often contains less water and more solid matter, including nutrients. So it doesn't really cost that much more, and is so much better for you. In addition buy brown rice, wholewheat bread or pasta or other wholefoods such as beans, lentils, nuts and wholegrains, which contain a full complement of nutrients.

Bake, boil, steam or steam-fry, instead of oil-frying

Frying food in oil or butter at high temperatures not only destroys essential nutrients, especially the fat-soluble antioxidant vitamins A and E, but also creates oxidants which have the power to damage body cells. Many dishes can be 'steam-fried' by adding a water-based sauce and steaming the con-tents of the dish (examples are given below). If you do fry food, use a tiny amount of butter or olive oil (not cold-pressed organic seed oil), fry for as short a time as possible, then add the sauce and cover the pan to allow the food to steam.

As a general guideline, eat:

- five servings of fresh fruit and vegetables daily, to include . . .
  - one serving of cruciferous vegetables (broccoli, cabbage, cauliflower, Brussels sprouts, kale)
  - one carrot, one sweet potato, some watercress or peas (high in carotenoids)
  - one 'berry' fruit portion, when in season (high in flavonoids)

- some soya produce, be it a glass of soya milk or some tofu, every other day

- carnivorous fish (salmon, tuna, herring, mackerel) three times a week

- one serving of quinoa twice a week (vegetarians should have more tofu and quinoa)

- a heaped tablespoon of ground seeds (sesame, sunflower, flax and pump-kin) or a tablespoon of an organic oil blend every day

- one clove of garlic a day

- one serving of shiitake mushrooms twice a week

A typical week's menu, for which recipes can be found on p. 188, might look like this:

Monday

BREAKFAST
Organic Cornflakes with Ground Seeds and Chopped Apple with
soya, rice or skimmed milk

LUNCH
Braised Tofu, Tahini and Watercress Rye Sandwich

DINNER
Grilled or Poached Salmon with Mashed Sweet Potato and Brussels
sprouts in a Hummus and Mushroom Sauce

Tuesday

BREAKFAST
Get Up and Go with Soya Milk and Banana

LUNCH
Sweet Potato and Carrot Soup

DINNER
Spicy Chickpea Pasta and a Green Salad

Wednesday

BREAKFAST
Oat or Millet flakes with Pear and Ground Seeds with soya, rice or
skimmed milk

LUNCH
Baked Potato with Tuna and Sweetcorn

DINNER
Buckwheat Noodles with Shiitake Mushrooms Thai Style
followed by Mixed Berries with Cashew Cream

Thursday

BREAKFAST
Get Up and Go with Soya Milk and Banana

LUNCH
Rainbow Root Salad

DINNER
Chestnut Hotpot with Quinoa

Friday

BREAKFAST
Scots Porridge with Banana and Seeds

LUNCH
Carrot Soup in the Raw and Oatcakes

DINNER
Vegetable Steam-fry *followed by* Berry Ice-cream

Saturday

BREAKFAST
Oat Muesli with fruit

LUNCH
Provençal Vegetables with Goat's Cheese Dressing

DINNER
Almond Mackerel with Cauliflower Cheese and Lemon Kale

Sunday

BREAKFAST
Scrambled Eggs with Smoked Salmon and Chives

LUNCH
Shiitake Mushrooms, Tofu and Vegetables *followed by* Berry Pie

DINNER
Quinoa Ratatouille

Each day, eat two pieces of fresh fruit, as snacks, mid-morning and mid-afternoon.

TWENTY-SEVEN

SUPPLEMENTS TO SURVIVE AND THRIVE IN THE TWENTY-FIRST CENTURY

The most common concern raised about taking supplements is people's intuitive feeling that, surely, we should be getting all the nutrients we need from a well-balanced diet? But is this really intuition, or cultural and political brain-washing? The first time I read such a statement was in a Health Education Council booklet that stated, 'As long as you eat a well-balanced diet you get all the vitamins and minerals you need'. There were no facts, no science to back it up. A shocking number of people – more than one in 10 – fail to achieve even the government's RDA level of vitamins and minerals, which is in fact a very low level indeed. These Recommended Daily Allowances are often no more than a fifth of optimal levels – and aren't even set for many essential nutrients and for any non-essential but beneficial phytochemicals.

If you look at the history of the evolution of different species it is clear that we all compete for nutrients. Those species who do well survive and evolve; those that do badly become extinct. With increasing ingenuity the survivors find out how to adapt to changing circumstances by changing their diet and lifestyle. Now, at the dawn of the twenty-first century, we have an uphill battle, faced with a barrage of antinutrients in food, water, air and household products. To survive or, rather, thrive in the twenty-first century we need more than a 'well-balanced diet'. We need to ensure an optimal intake of nutrients to help protect us from these unavoidable antinutrients and toxins, as well as to achieve our maximum potential as a human being.

You, as an individual, are evolving now – it's not something that happened in the past and then stopped. The same is true for humanity as a species. Everything we do affects not only us, but also the generations to come. Sigmund Freud based his whole concept of the human psyche on the existence of two instincts: to survive as an individual, and to survive as a species. Reading this book is an expression of these instincts working. Carl Jung added another dimension – the desire to reach one's fullest potential. Only with the fullest expression of who you are can you make the biggest difference to those around you.

Choosing an optimal diet, plus an appropriate supplement programme, is probably the most tangible and guaranteed investment you can make in yourself. Unlike life insurance policies, the benefits come after just weeks, and accumulate over months and years. Unlike health insurance policies, you get to experience health now, rather than insuring the best medical attention when you're on the way out. As one man said, 'Never mind if there's life after death. What I want is life before death.'

Supplementary Benefit

The following pages give advice on what to supplement on top of an optimal diet in order to thrive in the twenty-first century. I've also suggested extra nutrients and top-ups on others once you reach the age of fifty. There's nothing magical about fifty. Indeed, some of our bodies reach the biological age of fifty as early as thirty or as late as seventy.

The best route of all is to invest in a professional assessment of your nutrition needs from a qualified nutrition consultant. This really is essential if you have health problems that aren't responding to current treatment or are only controlled by drugs with undesirable long-term effects. (If you are currently on medication for a particular condition, please check with your doctor that there is no contra-indication for you to supplement any of these nutrients.) The Useful Addresses section tells you how to find a local nutrition consultant, trained at the Institute for Optimum Nutrition, who will be well versed in all the approaches covered in this book.

Supplements – Which, When and How?

The information given here is only a set of guidelines to help you to get into the ballpark of optimum nutrition. For fine-tuning, my book *The Optimum Nutrition Bible* shows you how to assess your own personal needs using the Optimum Nutrition Questionnaire. Many of these nutrients are provided in special formulas, or in complexes that cut down the number of tablets you take. I've grouped those that are most likely to appear together and indicated what kind of supplement to look for.

Since the right dose makes all the difference, you'll need to shop around and check out different formulas. Once again, *The Optimum Nutrition Bible* gives you detailed information on choosing the right supplements, deciphering the labels and finding your way round the extensive shelves of supplements in health food stores; or again, ideally, see a nutrition consultant who can work out your personal programme and tell you what is best for you. Alternatively, don't be afraid to ask a health food store assistant to look at this list and let you know what is the best way to meet your needs. Many stores have product advisers specifically trained to do so.

Also, don't expect miracles overnight. Nutrients take time to work. Many people feel better within six weeks and most within three months, which is the ideal length of time to commit yourself to a supplement programme. The real effect occurs when your body receives the right nutrients daily and, one by one, your body cells become fitter and healthier. You will notice the difference to your quality of life after two years. Since it takes seven years for virtually every cell in your body, including your bones, to be replaced, the long-term effect of optimum nutrition is a new and healthier you.

On the whole, take supplements with food – they *are* food. But a few nutrients are best absorbed on an empty stomach. For example, individual amino acids, such as glutamine or lysine, have to compete for absorption with other amino acids in protein-rich foods. So if you supplement these separately from food you'll absorb more.

Most nutrients contribute to the energy you'll need to produce during the day, so it's good to take them in the morning. But you'll make better use of supplements by spreading them throughout the day: for the very organised, across three meals is ideal. If you opt for twice a day the best time is breakfast and lunch, although working people may prefer breakfast and dinner to avoid having to take supplements to work. Probably the most practical, although not the ideal, way to take supplements is all in the morning. That's what I do when I'm travelling.

Side-effects

The side-effects of optimum nutrition are better energy, fewer colds, fewer infections, better skin and freedom from disease. However, if you ever experience nausea you are probably taking too many supplements and not enough food, since supplements need digestive juices to aid their absorption. In this event, simply spread out your supplements, taking equal amounts with each meal. If you suspect that something doesn't suit you, stop them all and reintroduce them one at a time at four-day intervals. Adverse reactions are almost always transient and very rare. Nothing I've covered in this book gets you anywhere near a toxic level of nutrients. Again, this subject is covered in full in *The Optimum Nutrition Bible*.

Daily Supplement Checklist

	Daily amount	Best form/source
Essential Supplements		
Vitamin A (retinol)	5000ius	
Betacarotene	5000ius	natural source, not synthetic
Vitamin C	2000mg	calcium or magnesium ascorbate
Vitamin E	300ius	d-alpha tocopherol with mixed tocopherols
Vitamin B1 (thiamine)	50mg	
Vitamin B2 (riboflavin)	50mg	
Vitamin B3 (niacin)	75mg	
Vitamin B6 (pyridoxine)	100mg	
Vitamin B12	10mcg	
Folic acid	200mcg	
Biotin	100mcg	
Calcium	300mg	citrate/ascorbate/amino acid chelate
Magnesium	150mg	citrate/ascorbate/amino acid chelate
Iron	10mg	citrate/ascorbate/amino acid chelate
Zinc	15mg	citrate/ascorbate/amino acid chelate
Manganese	5mg	citrate/ascorbate/amino acid chelate
Selenium	100mcg	selenomethionine or selenocysteine
Chromium	50mcg	picolinate or polynicotinate

All these can be provided in a high-potency multivitamin and mineral formula plus an antoxidant nutrient formula, plus an additional 1000mg vitamin C a day

	Daily amount	Best form/source
Optional supplements		
Gamma linolenic Acid (GLA)	150mg	Primrose oil or starflower oil
EPA and DHA	500mg	Fish oil or special algae

These can be provided as evening primrose oil or starflower oil capsules (for GLA), and as fish oil or algae capsules (for EPA/DHA), or from the diet in fish, seeds or their oils.

Pantothenic acid	an extra 300mg
Phosphatidyl choline	1000mg
or DMAE	500mg
Pyroglutamate	450mg

These can be provided in a brain food supplement.

Other optional supplements are blue-green algae, aloe vera, ginkgo biloba, 'green' powders from grasses and phytonutrient complexes which are sometimes supplied in advanced multivitamin formulas.

	Daily amount	Best form/source

Ideal additions to the above for the over-fifties

Vitamin C	an extra 1000mg
Vitamin E	an extra 300ius
DHA	an extra 300mg
Calcium	an extra 400mg
Magnesium	an extra 300mg

For all the complexity and detailed information in this book, the message remains simple. Disease is the result of our unsuccessful adaptation to the environment – an environment which we have rendered virtually unable to support a healthy life. Tomorrow's medicine will be about restoring this environment – through consciously reducing our exposure to antinutrients, improving our lifestyle, and fundamentally changing the food we eat. We are moving from a period of pharmaceutical medicine into the era of nutritional medicine. This is because it works better – nutrients are not alien to the body but part of its design. They help us to adapt successfully.

The emphasis will also shift towards genuine healthcare – the promotion of health rather than the treatment of disease. This was predicted by the great inventor Thomas Edison, who said in 1890, 'The doctor of the future will give no medicine but will interest his patients in the care of the human frame, diet and the cause and prevention of disease.' Tomorrow's medicine is for you – today. I wish you 100% health and a long, rewarding life in the new millennium.

RECIPES FOR THE
NEW MILLENNIUM

These recipes will enable you to put into action the sample weekly menu in Chapter 26. There's a shopping list at the end to help you find the right ingredients for a healthy diet.

Breakfasts

Get Up and Go with Soya Milk and Banana

SERVES 1

This is a breakfast drink made by blending skimmed milk or soya milk with a banana and a serving of Get Up and Go, a nutrient-rich powder containing complex carbohydrates, protein derived from quinoa, vitamins, minerals, sesame, sunflower and pumpkin seeds, oatgerm, oatbran and beneficial bacteria. Each serving provides the RDA of every known essential nutrient plus many more as yet without RDAs, from essential fatty acids to beneficial bacteria, a third of all the protein you need, plus complex carbohydrate, fibre and very little fat. It contains no sucrose, no additives, no animal products, no milk, no wheat and no yeast.

Each serving, with skimmed milk and a banana, provides fewer than 300 calories, making it ideal as part of a balanced low-calorie diet. It is nutritionally superior to any other breakfast choice and is totally suitable for adults and children alike. It is fine to have this for breakfast every day, if you choose. It is available in any good health food shop or, by mail order, from Higher Nature (see Directory of Supplement Manufacturers).

> 1 serving Get Up and Go
> 300ml (½ pint) skimmed milk *or* low-fat soya milk
> 1 banana

Put all the ingredients into a blender and blend until smooth. You can add a spoonful of ground sesame seeds, sunflower seeds and linseeds to top up those already in the powder, or a little cinnamon for flavour, and you could experiment with other fruits – try peaches, strawberries, blueberries, pears, mangoes etc.

Scots Porridge with Banana and Seeds

SERVES 1

On a cold winter's day nothing can be more warming than porridge. Oats contain special factors that are known to promote a healthy heart and arteries, and are full of fibre and complex carbohydrates.

300ml (½ pint) water
300ml (½ pint) soya milk *or* rice milk *or* oat milk
25g (1oz) porridge oats

To serve:
1 banana, sliced
Ground sunflower seeds, sesame seeds, *and* linseeds *or* pumpkin seeds

Put the water and half the milk in a pan and sprinkle in the oats. Bring to the boil and boil for just under five minutes, stirring all the time. Serve with the remaining soya milk, the banana and the ground seeds.

Oat Muesli with Fruit

SERVES 4

This recipe comes courtesy of the great chef Anton Mosimann. It is a real treat and a great way to start the weekend.

4 tablespoons rolled oats
1 tablespoon oat germ and bran

100ml (4fl.oz) soya milk, warmed
150g (5oz) plain yoghurt
2 tablespoons honey
2 tablespoons lemon juice
1 red apple, washed, cored and grated, but not peeled
1 green apple, washed, cored and grated, but not peeled
4 tablespoons (60ml) chopped hazelnuts
300g (10oz) berries, e.g. strawberries, raspberries, blueberries, sliced if necessary

To serve:
4 sprigs fresh mint
4–8 whole berries in perfect condition

Soak the rolled oats, oat germ and bran and soya milk together in a bowl for at least two hours. Stir in the yoghurt, honey and lemon juice, then add the apples and hazelnuts, followed by the berries just before serving. Garnish with the mint and whole berries.

Scrambled Eggs with Smoked Salmon and Chives

SERVES 1

While eggs are rather high in fats, as an occasional part of a balanced diet they are a good source of protein. Grain-fed, free-range chickens lay eggs richer in essential fats.

15g (½oz) butter
2 free-range eggs, beaten
1 tablespoon chopped parsley
50g (2oz) smoked salmon pieces, cut small
2 fresh chives, chopped
Lemon juice

To serve:
Wholewheat or whole rye toast

Melt the butter in a small pan, then add the eggs and parsley. Cook slowly, stirring constantly with a wooden spoon or spatula. Add the smoked salmon. Squeeze fresh lemon juice on top to taste, sprinkle with the chives, and serve on the toast.

Lunches

Braised Tofu, Tahini and Watercress Rye Sandwich

SERVES 1

Plain tofu needs flavour added, otherwise it's boring. You can buy marinated tofu pieces or smoked tofu, both of which have some flavour. Try it with tahini, a spread made from sesame seeds and their oil. Keep this in the fridge once opened.

½ can braised tofu, chopped
½ bunch watercress
1 dessertspoon tahini
2 slices rye bread

Spread tahini on both slices of bread, then add the tofu and watercress to make a sandwich.

Sweet Potato and Carrot Soup

SERVES 2

Sweet potatoes are rich in carotenoids and vitamin E. This simple soup takes only a few minutes to prepare and tastes delicious. An alternative to sweet potato is butternut squash.

4 medium sweet potatoes, peeled and chopped small
4 large carrots, chopped small
⅓ can coconut milk (400ml/14fl.oz can)
1 clove garlic, crushed
Black pepper

Boil the sweet potatoes and the carrots until soft in just enough water to cover them. Purée in a blender or mouli, then add the coconut milk, garlic and black pepper to taste.

Rainbow Root Salad

SERVES 4

This colourful combination of carrots, cabbage, parsnips and beetroot is more filling than you think. Go easy on the beetroot and parsnip as their strong taste can overpower the carrots.

    3 medium carrots, grated
    ¼ red cabbage, grated
    1 small parsnip, grated
    1 medium raw beetroot, grated
    2 tablespoons Essential Balance oil
    1 teaspoon Dijon mustard
    2 cloves garlic, crushed
    Lemon juice
    Parsley, finely chopped

Mix together all the root vegetables in a large salad bowl. Mix the oil, mustard, garlic and lemon juice to taste in a cup or jug. Add to the salad and toss or stir well together. Sprinkle the parsley over the top.

Carrot Soup in the Raw

SERVES 4

Ever had a hot, raw soup? This soup is made cold and then heated gently, which keeps all the vitamin and mineral content intact. It's also full of fibre. Don't overheat it.

    450g (1lb) carrots
    75g (3oz) ground almonds
    300ml (½ pint) skimmed milk or soya milk
    1 teaspoon vegetable stock concentrate, e.g. Vecon
    1 teaspoon dried mixed herbs

Place the carrots in a food processor and blend to a purée. Add the other ingredients and process until well combined. Warm the soup very gently in a pan.

Provençal Vegetables with Goat's Cheese Dressing

SERVES 4

This dish comes courtesy of Ursula Ferringo from her book *Real Fast Vegetarian Food* (Metro) and captures the flavours of Provence. Do be sure to use good goat's cheese, but not too strong or it might mask the taste of the vegetables. Serve the vegetables just warm so that the flavour of the dressing is absorbed.

    6 ripe tomatoes
    75g (3oz) mild to medium goat's cheese
    2 cloves garlic, roughly crushed
    4 tablespoons Essential Balance oil
    1 tablespoon lemon juice
    salt
    black pepper
    Handful of pine kernels
    100g (4oz) broccoli florets
    100g (4oz) French beans
    100g (4oz) mangetout
    2 small courgettes, thickly sliced

To make the dressing, put the tomatoes in a bowl, cover with boiling water for about 30 seconds, then plunge into cold water. Using a sharp knife, peel off the skins and then roughly chop the flesh, discarding the seeds. Put the tomatoes, goat's cheese, garlic, oil, lemon juice, salt and pepper in a food processor and blend until smooth. Spread the pine kernels on a baking tray and toast under the grill, turning them frequently (watch them like a hawk, for they easily burn). Set aside. In a large saucepan of boiling salted water, blanch the vegetables in batches until just tender but still very firm to the bite. Allow about 4–5 minutes for the broccoli, 4 minutes for the beans and 2 minutes for the mangetout and courgettes. Remove from the pan with a slotted spoon and drain each batch of vegetables well. To serve, pour the dressing over the vegetables and garnish with the pine kernels.

Shiitake Mushrooms, Tofu and Vegetables

SERVES 4

This dish is a great introduction to oriental cooking. The ingredients can easily be found in an oriental supermarket.

1 cube canned red fermented bean curd, mixed to a smooth paste in ½ cup water

300g (10oz) canned lotus roots, sliced to 6mm (¼ in) width

300g (10oz) canned bamboo roots

1 tablespoon olive oil *or* vegetable oil

4 cloves garlic, finely chopped

250g (8oz) shiitake mushrooms (if you can't get fresh, use dried and soak them)

1 teaspoon soya sauce

1 teaspoon sesame oil

1 teaspoon vegetable stock concentrate, e.g. Vecon

6 pieces of firm tofu, sliced to 12mm (½in) width

To serve:

Small bunch coriander leaves, finely chopped

2 spring onions, finely chopped

Rice *or* noodles

Put the bean mixture in a deep pan and quickly bring to the boil. Turn the heat down to medium, then add the lotus roots and bamboo roots and stir them in. Cook slowly for 3 minutes, cover and keep warm. Heat the oil in a pan on medium heat. Add the garlic and stir briefly. Add the mushrooms and stir for 2–3 minutes. Add the soya sauce and ½ teaspoon of the sesame oil. Reduce the heat, cover and cook for 2 minutes, then put aside and keep warm. Pour ½ cup water into a large pan, add the Vecon and bring to the boil. Add the remaining sesame oil and stir well. Gently add the tofu slices. Spoon the liquid over the tofu and cover the pan. Cook on a very low heat for 2 minutes. Now take a large plate, dish out the tofu in the centre and surround it with the lotus and bamboo roots. Pour the mushrooms and juice on top of the tofu. Garnish with coriander and spring onions and serve with rice or noodles.

Dinners

Grilled or Poached Salmon with Mashed Sweet Potato and Brussels Sprouts in a Hummus and Mushroom Sauce

SERVES 2

2 pieces salmon fillet *or* 2 salmon steaks

2 large sweet potatoes

Black pepper
250g (8oz) Brussels sprouts
250g (9oz) organic brown mushrooms *or* shiitake mushrooms
25g (1oz) butter
125g (4oz) hummus

Grill or poach the salmon (see any cookbook for instructions). Boil and mash the sweet potatoes, adding black pepper to taste. Boil or steam the Brussels sprouts for 5 minutes. Sauté the mushrooms in the butter for 2 minutes, then add a little water, cover and turn the heat down. Let them cook for 5 minutes until tender and juicy. Purée the mushrooms and add the hummus. Add the Brussels sprouts and serve, accompanied by the salmon and the mashed sweet potatoes.

Spicy Chickpea Pasta

SERVES 4

This recipe comes courtesy of ION nutritionist and chef Anne Gains, and the delicious sauce is equally good with pasta, buckwheat noodles or rice. Chickpeas are an excellent source of protein. If using pasta, make sure you get wholemeal.

1–2 tablespoons olive oil
1 large onion, chopped
1 large parsnip, chopped
1 large carrot, chopped
2 cloves garlic, crushed
1 aubergine, cut into chunks
½ teaspoon mild chilli powder (optional)
1 teaspoon ground cumin
1 teaspoon ground coriander
425g (15oz) canned tomatoes *or* fresh tomatoes, chopped
300ml (½ pint) vegetable stock
100g (4oz) mushrooms, quartered
250g (8oz) broccoli, cut into florets
100g (4oz) chickpeas, soaked, cooked and drained, *or* canned (pre-cooked)
425g (15oz) wholemeal pasta shapes *or* spaghetti

Heat the oil in a large pan and add the onion, parsnip, carrot, garlic and aubergine. Cook for 5 minutes, stirring all the time. Add the spices and mix thoroughly before adding the tomatoes and stock. Bring to the boil, then reduce the heat and simmer slowly for 15 minutes. Add the mushrooms, broccoli and chickpeas and continue cooking for 5 minutes, adding a little more stock if necessary to make a good sauce. Meanwhile, cook the pasta in plenty of water until *al dente*, drain and serve with the sauce, sprinkling with a little extra ground coriander. Serve with a fresh green salad dressed with 1 tablespoon of Essential Balance oil.

Buckwheat Noodles with Shiitake Mushrooms Thai Style

SERVES 2

Buckwheat is a wheat-free food with a good protein content. Most buckwheat noodles also contain wheat and these are easier to cook than pure buckwheat noodles, which fall apart if cooked too long. They are best boiled for 5 minutes, then drained, then boiled again. A specific mix of oriental herbs and spices is available in packets from many supermarkets.

    2 cloves garlic, chopped
    25g (1oz) butter
    100g (3½ oz) shiitake mushrooms, chopped or sliced
    1 green pepper, thinly sliced
    2 carrots, thinly sliced lengthways in 5cm (3inch) lengths
    100g (3½ oz) marinated tofu pieces
    100g (3½ oz) broccoli, cut into florets
    1 teaspoon Thai spices plus 2 tablespoons coconut milk *or* 1 tablespoon soy sauce
    200g (7oz) buckwheat noodles

Sauté the garlic in the butter for 3 minutes, then add the mushrooms and fry briefly before adding the rest of the vegetables, the tofu, spices and coconut milk and enough water for the ingredients to steam-fry. Cover and turn down the heat. Cook the buckwheat noodles in boiling water for 8 minutes. Drain and serve with the mushroom mixture.

Chestnut Hotpot with Quinoa

SERVES 4

Chestnuts are the lowest-fat nuts by a long way, so enjoy yourself in the chestnut season. Out of season you can use dried chestnuts, which simply need soaking overnight (and are much easier to prepare!).

150g (5oz) dried *or* 250g (8oz) fresh chestnuts
1 medium onion, sliced
2 cloves garlic, crushed
25g (1oz) butter
250g (8oz) carrots, sliced
250g (8oz) potatoes, sliced
250g (8oz) swede, sliced
250g (8oz) turnip, sliced
300ml (½ pint) vegetable stock
Black pepper
375g (2oz) quinoa

If using dried chestnuts, soak overnight. Sauté the onion and garlic in the butter. Slice all the vegetables and add to the pan with the stock, pepper and chestnuts. Simmer very gently for 30–40 minutes until the chestnuts are just soft. Boil the quinoa in 900ml (1½ pints) water for 15 minutes, or until soft, and drain.

Vegetable Steam-fry

This method of cooking makes endless varieties of delicious main meals in no more than 10 minutes. You need a shallow, thick-based pan with a tight-fitting lid. Select from carrots, broccoli, cauliflower, mangetout, broad beans, water chestnuts, almonds, organic or shiitake mushrooms, bamboo shoots, green and red peppers, courgettes and tofu. Wash the vegetables and cut into pieces. Put a dab of olive oil in your chosen pan and sauté the vegetables for 1 minute. Add one of the following sauces, if liked, and steam for 5 minutes. Serve with brown rice, quinoa or buckwheat noodles.

CHINESE: Add 1 teaspoon grated ginger and 2 cloves crushed garlic to the pan with the sautéed vegetables. After 1 minute add 2 tablespoons soy sauce and 4 tablespoons water, a 227g can sliced bamboo shoots, drained, and a 227g can whole water chestnuts, drained.

THAI: To the sautéed vegetables add 100ml (4fl.oz) coconut milk and your choice of Thai spices.

MEXICAN: To the sautéed vegetables add some Discovery Mexican Spice Sauce, diluted with water. Use as much or as little as you like.

MEDITERRANEAN: Add to the sautéed vegetables 2 cloves garlic, crushed, 1 level tablespoon mixed herbs, 50g (2oz) black olives, chopped, and some Whole Earth Organic Spaghetti Sauce.

Almond Mackerel with Cauliflower Cheese and Lemon Kale

SERVES 2

Mackerel is rich in essential fats, as are almonds. Kale is an excellent source
of many nutrients, including calcium. This recipe makes it all taste great, too.

    2 medium mackerel fillets
    125g (4oz) sliced almonds
    1 teaspoon dried mixed herbs
    Olive oil
    Large knob of butter
    1 tablespoon maize flour
    250ml (⅓ pint) soya milk
    250g (8oz) soya cheese, grated
    Black pepper
    1 medium cauliflower
    450g (1lb) curly kale
    3 cloves garlic, crushed
    Juice of ½ lemon
    Soy sauce

Wash and dry the mackerel fillets. Place on a board, skin side down, and scat-
ter with the herbs and almonds. Preheat the oven to 375°F/190°C/gas mark
5. Oil a baking dish with olive oil. Add the fish, sprinkle with lemon juice, a
little oil and pepper, and bake for 20–30 minutes. Make a white sauce in the
usual way, using maize flour (unrefined cornflour), butter and soya milk. Add
the soya cheese and black pepper. Steam the cauliflower until tender but still
with a little 'bite'. Pour the sauce on top and place in the oven to keep hot.
Sauté the garlic in a little olive oil in a 'steam-fry' pan (see p.197). Add the
kale and stir for 2 minutes just to generate heat. Mix together the remaining
lemon juice and soy sauce, add the same volume of water, and add the mixture to the kale. This should instantly steam. Cover the pan and cook for 4
minutes, then serve accompanied by the mackerel and cauliflower cheese.

Quinoa Ratatouille

SERVES 2

Ratatouille is a Provençal dish using vegetables grown in the South of France.

1 tablespoon olive oil
1 onion, chopped
2 cloves garlic, chopped
2 courgettes, thickly sliced
1 aubergine, cubed
1 green pepper, sliced
1 teaspoon dried mixed herbs
2 tomatoes, skinned (see p. 193) and roughly chopped
320g (6oz) quinoa

Sauté the onion and garlic briefly in the oil, then add the courgettes followed by the aubergine and the green pepper, stirring all the time. Then add a little water and the herbs. Finally add the tomatoes plus some more water if needed, so that the vegetables are cooking in their own juice. Turn down the heat, cover the pan and cook for 15 minutes. Boil the quinoa in 600ml (1 pint) water for 15 minutes. Drain and serve with the ratatouille.

Desserts

Summer Pudding

SERVES 4

Eat berries fresh when in season, and canned in apple juice when they're not. Most supermarkets stock berries in apple juice. These can be eaten on cereal, in fruit salads or in the following recipes, while the juice can be drunk as an all-round tonic. The summer pudding recipe can be turned into an Autumn Pudding by using cooked blackberries, apples and dried fruits instead of summer berries.

4–6 slices rye bread, crusts removed
1 punnet strawberries, quartered
2 punnets raspberries
1 punnet blueberries or blackcurrants
300–350ml (10–12fl.oz) orange juice
1–2 tablespoons maple syrup or honey

Combine the berries, orange juice and syrup or honey in a bowl and leave to stand for 1 hour. Line a 600ml (1 pint) basin with most of the bread, spoon in the fruit and juice, then make a lid with the remaining bread. Place a saucer on top, weighed down with a heavy can and leave overnight in the fridge. Turn out on to a plate to serve.

Mixed Berries with Cashew Cream

SERVES 4

450g (1lb) mixed berries
125g (4oz) 1 cup ground cashew nuts
Soya milk *or* honey

Wash the berries and divide among four small bowls. Blend the cashew nuts with a little water. Add soya milk or honey to taste, pour the cashew cream over the berries, and serve.

Berry Ice-cream

Dairy-free vanilla ice-cream. Mixed berries of your choice. Reserve a few of the best-looking berries and put the rest in an electric blender to make a sauce. Sprinkle the reserved berries on the ice-cream, then pour the berry sauce over the top.

Snacks and Drinks

For snacks have two pieces of fresh fruit a day between meals, perhaps with a few almonds. If you're really hungry eat a couple of oatcakes or a raw carrot with some hummus.

Drink water, water with a touch of blackcurrant and apple concentrate, or diluted fruit juice.

Shopping List

These foods are readily found in health food stores, and some can be obtained in supermarkets:

Organic cornflakes, oatflakes, millet flakes
Braised, marinated, smoked or plain firm tofu
Tahini
Buckwheat noodles (soba)
Dried shiitake mushrooms
Quinoa
Dairy-free ice-cream
Soya milk
Rice milk (Rice Dream)
Oatcakes (sugar-free)
Vegetable stock (Vecon or Bouillon)
Seeds: sesame, sunflower, pumpkin and linseeds
Cold-pressed oil blends from the above seeds, such as Essential Balance
(distributed by Higher Nature: see Directory of Supplement Manufacturers) or
Udo's Choice
Coconut milk
Discovery Mexican Spice Sauce
Thai spices
Amoy sliced bamboo shoots in water
Amoy whole water chestnuts in water
Whole Earth Organic Spaghetti Sauce
Cauldron Foods marinated Tofu Pieces

Most of your food comes from the greengrocer, organic when possible:
Lots of fresh fruit and vegetables

RECOMMENDED READING

The following books and publications will help you to dig deeper into the subjects covered in this book.

GENERAL
Holford, Patrick, *The Optimum Nutrition Bible*, Piatkus, 1997

CHAPTERS 3 and 5
Capra, Fritjof, *The Web of Life*, HarperCollins, 1996

CHAPTER 7
Cannon, Geoffrey, *Superbug*, Virgin, 1995

CHAPTER 8
Holford, Patrick, and Pfeiffer, Carl, *Mental Health and Mental Illness*, ION Press, 1996

CHAPTER 9
Colborn, Theo, Myers and Dumanoski, *Our Stolen Future*, Little Brown, 1996
Cadbury, Deborah, *The Feminisation of Nature*, Hamish Hamilton, 1997

CHAPTERS 10 and 11
Neil, Kate, *Balancing Hormones Naturally*, ION Press, 1995
Lee, William, *What Your Doctor Didn't Tell You About Menopause*, Warner, 1996

CHAPTER 12
Passwater, Richard, *Cancer Prevention and Nutritional Therapies*, Keats, 1993
Lane, William, *Sharks Don't Get Cancer*, Avery, 1992

CHAPTER 13
Pauling, Linus, *Unified Theory on the Cause and Treatment of Cardiovascular Disease*, ION video, 1995

CHAPTER 14
Holford, Patrick, *Say No to Arthritis*, ION Press, 1993
Bland, Jeffrey, *The 20-Day Rejuvenation Diet Program*, Keats, 1997

CHAPTER 15
Meek, Jennifer, *Boost Your Immune System*, ION Press, 1996

CHAPTER 16
Holford, Patrick, *The New Fatburner Diet*, ION Press, 1995

CHAPTER 17
The 20-Day Rejuvenation Diet Program (see Chapter 14)

CHAPTER 19
Carper, Jean, *Stop Ageing Now*, Thorsons, 1997
Holford, Patrick, and Barlow, Philip, *How to Protect Yourself from Pollution*, ION Press, 1990

CHAPTER 23
Lombard, Jay, *Brain Wellness Plan*, Kensington Books, 1997

CHAPTER 24
Dean, Ward, and Morgenthaler, John, *Smart Drugs and Nutrients*, B&J Publications, 1990
Dean, Ward, Morgenthaler, John, and Fowkes, Steven, *Smart Drugs 2 – The Next Generation*, Health Freedom Publications, 1993

REFERENCES

The references listed here relate to the main studies referred to, and numbered, in the text. These represent a fraction of the scientific literature used to compile this book. Those readers who wish to dig deeper are advised to access the scientific literature held on file at the Institute for Optimum Nutrition, whose staff can carry out literature and library searches on any topics of interest (see the last page of this book).

1. Department of Health, personal communication, 1997. Also see *Health of the Nation*, HMSO report

2. Professor Sir Carter D – reported in *Daily Mail*, November 23, 1996 p.6

3. See ref 2 above

4. *British National Formulary*. The British Medical Association and Royal Pharmaceutical Society of Great Britain. Bath Press 1997

5. Dr Eric Raps – reported in the *Daily Mail* April 17, 1997 p.29

6. Youcha G. 'The cortisone dilemma.' *Science Digest*, Jan 1982:42–44

7. Brooks P et al. 'NSAIDS and osteoarthritis – help or hindrance?' *J Rheumatol* 1982;9:3–5

8. Pelter A. 'Tryptophan – The hidden truth.' *Optimum Nutrition Magazine*, Summer 1990;3.2:12

9. Bland J. 'Rejuvenation – A "Do it yourself project".' *Health Comm. Inc.* 1997

10. Davis MK et al. 'Infant feeding and childhood cancer.' *Lancet* 1988;2:365–368

11. Saarinen U. 'Prolonged breast feeding as prophylaxis for recurrent otitis media.' *Acta Paediat Scand* 1982; 71:567–571

12. Freedman R et al. 'Behavioral treatment of menopausal hot flushes: Evaluation by ambulatory monitoring.' *Am J obst Gyn* 1992;167:436–439

13. Cheraskin E. 'Medical (not health) care costs are rising . . . stupid!' *J Advanc in Med* 1994;7(4):223–230

14. Zusenq S et al. 'Determination of E-rosette forming lymphocytes in aged subjects with Taichiquan exercise.' *Int J Sports Med* 1989;10:217–219

15. Chandra R. 'Effect of vitamin and trace element supplementation on immune responses and infection in elderly subjects.' *Lancet* 1992;340:1124–1127

16. Wiley R et al. 'Isometric exercise training lowers resting blood pressure.' *Med Sci Sports Exercise* 1992; 24:749–754

17. Hemilia et al. 'Vitamin C and the common cold: A retrospective analysis of Chalmers' review.' *J Am College Nutrition* 1992;14(2):116–123

18. Manson J et al. 'A Prospective Study of Antioxidant Vitamins and Incidence of Coronary Heart Disease in Women.' *Circulation* 1991;84:4:11–546

19. Risch H et al. 'Dietary factors and the incidence of cancer of the stomach.' *Am J Epidemiol* 1985;122:947–959

20. You W et al. *J Natl Cancer Inst.* 18 Jan 1989;81(2):162–164
Dorant E et al. 'Consumption of onions and reduced risk of stomach carcinoma.' *Gastroenterology* 1996;110:12–20

21. 'Food, Nutrition and the Prevention of Cancer: A Global Perspective, World Cancer Research Fund 1997' Pub American Institute for Cancer Research, Washington DC

22. Shekelle R et al. 'Dietary vitamin A and rise of cancer in the Western Electric Study.' *Lancet* 1981 Nov 28;2:185–1190

23. Cannon G. 'Superbug.' Virgin Publishing. 1995

24. Pinner R et al. 'Trends in infectious diseases mortality in the United States.' *JAMA,* January 17, 1996;275(3):189–193
The Health of Adult Britain 1841–1994, Office of National Statistics

25. *Daily Mail* Tuesday, April 15, 1997. p.11

26. *New Scientist* 17 Dec 1994

27. Little P. 'Open randomised trial of prescription strategies in the management of sore throats.' *BMJ* 1977; 314:722

28. Harakeh S et al. 'Suppression of human immunodeficiency virus replication by ascorbate in chronically and acute infected cells.' *Proc Natl Acad Sci* Sept 1990;87:7245–7249

29. Godfrey J et al. 'Zinc for treating the common cold: review of all clinical trials since 1984.' *Altern Ther* 1996;2(6):63–72

30. Jaffe R et al. 'The biochemical-immunology window: a molecular view of psychiatric case management.' *Int Clin Nut Rev* 1992;12(1):9–26
Osmond H et al. 'Massive niacin treatment in schizophrenia.' *Lancet* 10 February 1962;316–320

31. Holford P and Pfeiffer C. 'Mental Health & Illness.' ION Press 1996:154–155

32. Birmingham et al. *Int J Eat Disord* 1994;15(3):251–255

33. Schoenthaler S 'The northern California diet – behaviour program: An empirical evaluation of 3000 incarcerated juveniles in Stanislaus County Juvenile Hall.' *Int J Biosocial Res* 1983;5(2):99–106

34. Godfrey P et al. 'Enhancement of recovery from psychiatric illness by methylfolate.' *Lancet* 1990;336:392–395

35. Smith K et al. 'Relapse of depression after rapid depletion of tryptophan.' *Lancet* March 29, 1997;349:915–919

36. Hartman E et al. 'Hypnotic effects of L-tryptophan.' *Arch Gen Psych* 31 Sept 1974

37. Gesch B. 'Natural Justice: A pilot study in evaluating and responding to criminal behaviour as an environmental phenomenon; The South Cumbria (England) Alternative Sentencing Options (SCASO) Project.' *Int J Biosocial Med Res*

38. Smith K et al. 'Relapse of depression after rapid depletion of Tryptophan.' *Lancet* March 29,1997;349:915–919

39. (as for 38)

40. Freur J et al. *Am J Epidemiol* 1992;136:1423

41. Wolff M, interviewed for Horizon, January 1996 (see also Ref 44)

42. Carlsen E et al. 'Evidence for decreasing semen quality during the past 50 years.' *Brit Med J* 1992;305:609–612

43. Ostrerline A. 'Diverging trends in incidence and mortality of testicular cancer in Denmark' 1943–1982. *Brit J of Cancer* 1986;53:501–505

44. Report of Cancer Incidence and Prevalence Projections, East Anglian Cancer Intelligence Unit, Department of Community Medicine, University of Cambridge, June 1997, Macmillan Cancer Relief

45. Campbell D et al. 'Cryptochidism in Scotland.' *BMJ* 1987

46. Matlai P et al. 'Trends in congenital malformations of the external genitalia.' *Lancet* 1985; letter p.108

47. Herbst A et al. *New England J Med* 1971;284:878–881

48. Gill W et al. 'Effects on human males of in utero exposure to exogenous sex hormones.' *Toxicity of Hormones in Perinatal Life* 1988, T Miri and H Nagasawa (eds), CRC Press

49. Chang K-J et al. 'Influences of percutaneous administration of estradiol and progesterone on human breast epithelial cell cycle in vivo.' *Fertility and Sterility* April 1995;63(4):785

50. Bergkvist L et al. 'The risk of breast cancer after estrogen and estrogen-progestin replacement.' *N Engl J Med* 1989;32:293–297

51. Colditz G et al. 'The use of estrogen and progestins and the risk of breast cancer in postmenopausal women.' *N Engl J Med* 1995;332:1589–93

52. Rogriguez C et al. 'Estrogen replace-ment therapy and fatal ovarian cancer.' *Am J Epidemiology* 1995;141(9):828–835

53. Messina M. 'The role of soy products in reducing risk of cancer.' *J of National Cancer Institute* 1991;83:541–546

54. Troll W. 'Soybean diet lowers breast tumour incidence in irradiated rats.' *Carcinogenesis* 1980;1:469–472

55. Barnes S. 'Soybeans inhibit mammary tumor growth in models of breast cancer.' *Mutagens and Carcinogens in Diet* 1990, M Pariza (ed) New York: Wiley

56. Horribin D. 'Gamma linolenic acid: An intermediate in essential fatty acid metabolism with potential as an ethical pharmaceutical and as a food.' *Rev Contemp Pharmacother* 1990;1:1–45

57. Springford M, Truman L, ION Research Project 1996

58. Mohr P et al. *Brit J Cancer* 1996;73:1552–1555

59. 'Alternatives in Health,' June/July 1995 (Surrey University Fertility study)

60. Campbell B & Ellison P. 'Menstrual variation in salivary testosterone among regularly cycling women.' *Hormone Research* 1992;37:132–136

61. Cumming R et al. *Am J Epidemiol* 1997;145:926–34

62. Allen L et al. 'Protein-induced hypercalcuria: A longer term study.' *Am J Clin Nutrition* 1979;32:741–749

63. Anand C et al. 'Effect of protein intake on calcium balance of young men given 500mg calcium daily.' *J of Nutrition* 1974;104:695–700

64. Katiyar S et al. 'Protective effects of silymarin against photocarcinogenesis in a mouse skin model.' *J Natl Cancer Inst* 1997;8(98):556–566

65. Cadbury D. 'The Feminisation of Nature.' Hamish Hamilton Pub. 1997;180–183

66. Basu T et al. 'Plasma vitamin A in patients with bronchial carcinoma.' *Brit J of Cancer* 1976;33(1):119–121

67. Bond G et al. 'Dietary vitamin A and lung cancer: Results of a case-control study among chemical workers.' *Nutrition and Cancer* 1987; 9(2&3):109–121

68. Stitch H et al. 'Response of oral leuko-plakias to the administration of vitamin A.' *Cancer Letters* 1988; 40(1):93–101

69. Pauling L and Cameron R. Proceeding of National Academy of Sciences. 1976;73(10):3685–9

70. Murata A and Morishige F. International Conference on Nutrition, Taijin, China, 1981. Report in *Medical Tribune* Jul 22, 1981

71. Wald N et al. 'Plasma retinol, beta-carotene and vitamin E levels in relation to future risk of breast cancer.' *Brit J Cancer* 1984;49:321–324

72. *Int J Cancer* 1996;65:140–144

73. Salonen J. 'Risk of cancer in relation to serum concentrations of selenium and vitamins A and E.' *Brit Med J* 1985;290:417–20

74. Clark L et al. 'Effects of selenium supplementation for cancer prevention in patients with carcinoma of the skin.' *JAMA* 1996;276(24):1957–1963

75. Hirayama T. 'A large scale cohort study on cancer risks by diet – with special reference to the risk reducing effects of green-yellow vegetables consumption.' Princess Takamatsu Symp 1985;16:41–53

76. 'Food, Nutrition and the Prevention of Cancer: A Global Perspective, World Cancer Research Fund 1997' Pub American Institute for Cancer Research, Washington DC

77. See ref 76 – Chapter 4.10 pp.238–242

78. Shekelle R et al. 'Dietary vitamin A and risk of cancer in the Western Electric Study.' *Lancet* 1981 (Nov 28);2:1185–90

79. Peters R et al. 'Cancer causes and control.' 1992;3:457–473

80. Uauy-Dagach R and Valenzuela A. 'Marine oils: the health benefits of n-3 fatty acids.' *Nutr Rev* 1996;54(11):S102–S108 'Meeting probes n-3 fatty acids' medical role.' *Inform* 1997;8(2):176–180

81. Evans B et al. 'Inhibition of 5a-reductase in genital skin fibroblasts and prostate tissue by dietary lignans and isoflavonoids.' *J Endocrinol* 1995;147:295–302

82. Food, Nutrition and the Prevention of Cancer: a global perspective.' World Cancer Research Fund, 1997

83. Holford P. 'Alcohol – The Whole Truth.' Optimum Nutrition, Spring 1997;10.2

84. 'Sharks Don't Get Cancer,' W Lane, L Cormac, Pub Avery, New York 1992

85. Pauling L and Rath M. 'A unified theory of human cardiovascular disease leading the way to the abolition of this disease as a cause for human mortality.' *J Orthomolecular Med* 1992;7(1):5–12

86. McCarron D. 'Role of adequate dietary calcium intake in the prevention and management of salt-sensitive hypertension.' *Am J Clin Nutr* 1997;65(2S):712S–716S
Osborne C et al. 'Evidence for the relationship of calcium to blood pressure.' *Nutr Rev* 1996;54(12):365–381
Whelton P et al. 'Effects of oral potassium of blood pressure.' *JAMA* 1997;2777(20):1624–1632
Dyckner T. *Brit Med J* 1983;286:1847–49

87. Cannon M et al. 'The effect of combined micronutrient supplementation on blood pressure.' 1990, ION library, London.

88. Altura B. 'Magnesium in cardiovascular biology.' *Scientific American* May/June 1995;28–35

89. Stephens N et al. 'Randomised controlled trial of vitamin E in patients with coronary disease: Cambridge Heart Antioxidant Study (CHAOS).' *Lancet* March 23, 1996;347

90. *New Eng J Med* May 20, 1993:1444–1449
New Eng J Med May 20, 1993:1450–1455

91. *Biomedical and Clinical Aspects of Coenzyme Q*, Ed. Folkers K, Yamamura Y, pub. Elsevier Science Publishers BV, Amsterdam, 1986

92. See 91

93. See 91

94. Arnold et al, *Science* 7 June 1996

95. Nijhoff W et al. 'Effects of consumption of Brussels sprouts on intestinal and lumphocytic glutathione S-transferase in humans.' *Carcinogenesis* 1995; 16(9):2125–2128

96. Kaufman. *J Am Geriatrics Ass* 1955;3:927

97. Gupta V et al. 'Chemistry and Pharmacology of Gum Resin of Boswellia Serrata.' *Indian Drugs* 1986;24(5):221–231

98. 'Curcumnoids – the active principles from Turmeric root.' Sabinsa Corporation.

99. Belch et al. *Am Rheum Dis* 1988;47:96–104

100. Kremer et al. *Lancet* 1985;1:184–187
Sperling. *Med World News* July 14, 1986
van der Tempel. *Ann Rheum Dis* 1990;49:76–80
Kremer et al. *Arthr & Rheum* 1990;33(6):810–822
Nielson et al. *Eur J Clin Investig* 1992;22:687–691

101. Jungeblut C. 'Inactivation of poliomyelitis virus by crystalline vitamin C (ascorbic acid).' *J of Experimental Med* 1935;62:517–521

102. Itzhaki et al. 'Herpes simplex virus type 1 in brain and risk of Alzheimer's disease.' *Lancet* 1997;349:241–244

103. Levander O et al. 'Vitamin E and selenium: contrasting and interacting nutritional determinants of host resistance to parasitic and viral infections.' *Int Antiviral News* 1996;4(5):84–86

104. Harakeh S & Jariwalla R et al. 'Suppression of human immunodeficiency virus replication by ascorbate in chronically and acute infected cells.' *Proc Natl Acad Sci* Sept 1990;87:7245–7249

105. Mumcuolglu M. 'Inhibition of Several Strains of Influenza Virus in vitro and Reduction of Symptoms by an elderberry extract during an outbreak of Influenza B Panama.' *J Alt & Comp Med* 1995;1(4):361–369

106. Reaven G. 'Role of insulin resistance in human disease.' *Diabetes* 1988;37:1595–1607

107. Anderson R. 'Chromium nutrition in the elderly,' RR Watson (ed): *The Handbook of Nutrition in the Aged* Boca Raton, FL, CRC, 1993;385–392

108. Morris B et al. 'Correlations between abnormalities in chromium and glucose metabolism in a group of diabetics.' *Clin Chem* 1988;34:1525–1526

109. Urberg M et al. 'Hypo-cholesterolemic effects of nicotinic acid and chromium supplementation.' *J Fam Pract* 1988;27:603–606

110. Davies S et al. 'Age-related decreases in chromium levels in 51,665 hair, sweat and serum samples from 40,872 patients – implications for the prevention of cardiovascular disease and type II diabetes mellitus.' *Metabolism* 1997;46(5):1–4

111. Riales R et al. 'Effects of chromium chloride supplementation on glucose tolerance and serum lipids including high density lipoprotein of adult men.' *A J Clin Nut* 1981;34:2670–2678
Abraham AS et al. 'The effects of chromium supplementation on serum glucose and lipids in patients with and without non-insulin-dependent diabetes.' *Metabolism* 1992;41:768
Glinsmann W et al. 'Effects of trivalent chromium on glucose tolerance.' *Metabolism* 1966;15:510–515
Levine R et al. 'Effects of oral chromium supplementation on the glucose tolerance of elderly human subjects.' *Metabolism* 1968;17:114–124

112. Enstrom J and Pauling L. 'Mortality among health-conscious elderly Californians.' *Proc Natl Sci* 1982;79:6023–6027

113. Paterson C 'Lead versus Health,' 1983:p.21 Pub. Wiley, London

114. US News and World Report 20 Feb 1989;106(7):77(2)

115. 'The Great British Sperm Disaster,' *Optimum Nutrition* 1996;9.2:49

116. Rea W. *Chemical Sensitivity, Boca Raton* CRC Press

117. Holford P 'Crime-nourishment or punishment?' *Optimum Nutrition* 1995;7.3:38
Gesch B. 'Natural Justice.' A pilot study in evaluating and responding to criminal behaviour as an environmental phenomenon: The South Cumbria (England) Alternative Sentencing Options (SCASO) project. *Int J Boisocial Med Res* 1995;12,1:41–68

118. Virkunnen M. *Neuropsychobiology* 1982;3:35–40 and 8:30–34

119. Schoenthaler S 'The northern California diet-behaviour program: An empirical evaluation of 3000 incarcerated juveniles in Stanislaus County Juvenile Hall.' *Int J Biosocial Res* 1983;5(2):99–106

120. Schauss G. 'Comparative hair mineral analysis results of 21 elements, in a random selected behaviourally 'normal' 19–59 year old population and violent adult offenders.' *Int J of Biosocial Research* 1981;1(2):21–41

121. Schoenthaler S et al. 'Controlled trial of vitamin-mineral supplementation on intelligence and brain function.' *Person Individ Diff* 1991;12(4):343–350
Schoenthaler S et al. 'Controlled trial of vitamin-mineral supplementation: Effects on intelligence and performance.' *Person Individ Diff* 1991;12(4):351–362

122. Menzies E. 'Disturbed children: The role of food and chemical sensitivities.' *Nutr Health* 1984;3:39–45

123. Gesch B. 'Natural Justice.' A pilot study in evaluating and responding to criminal behaviour as an environmental phenomenon: The South Cumbria (England) Alternative Sentencing Options (SCASO) project. *Int J Biosocial Med Res* 1995;12(1):41–68

124. Itzhaki R et al. *Lancet* 1997; 349:241–44

125. Levander O et al. *Proc Nutr Soc* 1995;54(2):475–487

126. *N Engl J Med* 1997;336:1216–22

127. Hoffman A et al. *Lancet* 1997 Jan 18;349:151

128. Amaducci L. *Psychopharmacol Bull* 1988;24(10):130–134

129. Ward D and Morgenthaler J. 'Smart Drugs & Nutrients.' B&J Publications. 1990:42–43

130. Pilch H et al. 'Piracetam elevates muscarinic cholinergic receptor density in the frontal cortex of aged but not of young mice.' *Psychopharmacology* 1988;94:74–8

131. Bartus RT et al. 'Profound effects of combining choline and piracetam on memory enhancement and cholinergic function in aged rats.' *Neurobiology of Aging* 1981;2:105–111

132. Morgan A. *Int J Vit Nutr Res* 1975;45:448–462

133. Benton D. 'Effect of vitamin and mineral supplementation on intelligence of a sample of school children.' *Lancet* Jan 23, 1988

134. Schoenthaler S et al. 'Controlled trial of vitamin-mineral supplementation: Effects on intelligence and performance.' *Person Individ Diff* 1991;12(4):351–362

135. Snowden W. *Person Individ Diff* 1997;22(1):131–134

136. Ward D and Morgenthaler J. *Smart Drugs II* Health Freedom Publishing 1993

137. Crook T et al. 'Effects of phosphatidylserine in age-associated memory impairment.' *Neurology* 1991;41(5):644–649

138. *The Ultimate Nutrient – Glutamine* Shabert J et al. Avery Publications. 1994

139. Bland J. 'Effect of orally consumed aloe vera juice on gastrointestinal function in normal humans.' *Prevention* 1995; Pub. Rodale Press USA

140. Masquelier J. 'Pycnogenols: Recent advances in the therapeutic activity of procyanidins.' *J Medicinal Plan Research* 1980;7:243–256

141. See Ref 76 & 77

142. Nijhoff W et al. 'Effects of Consumption of Brussels sprouts on intestinal and lymphatic glutathione S-transferase in humans.' *Carcinogenesis* 1995;16(9):2125–2128

143. You W et al. *J Natl Cancr Inst* 18 Jan 1989;81(2):162–164

144. Steinmetz et al. *Am J Epid* 1994;139(1):1–15

145. Carper J. *Stop Ageing Now* p.162 & 325, pub Thorsons, 1997

146. Sofroniou P. *Superfoods* Optimum Nutrition, Summer 1993;6(2):48–54

USEFUL ADDRESSES

British Society of Nutritional and Environmental Medicine
The organisation for medical doctors working with allergies (including chemical sensitivities) and nutritional problems. Full members are all doctors; associate membership and other categories exist for related professions. The Society holds regular meetings and publishes the *Journal of Nutritional and Environmental Medicine*. For further information (including a list of practitioners) please write to Mrs I. Mansell, PO Box 28, Totton, Southampton SO40 2ZA (tel: 01703 812124; fax: 01703 813912).

Institute for Optimum Nutrition (ION)
ION offers personal consultations with qualified nutrition consultants and runs courses including the one-day Optimum Nutrition Workshop, the Homestudy Course and the three-year Nutrition Consultants' Diploma course. It also has a Directory of Nutrition Consultants (£2) which will help you find a nutrition consultant in your area. For details send an sae to: ION, Blades Court, Deodar Road, London SW15 2NU (tel: 0181 877 9993; fax: 0181 877 9980). (See also p. 216).

Laboratory tests
All the tests mentioned in this book, can be undertaken by laboratories through qualified nutrition consultants and doctors. Find a nutrition consultant by contacting ION.

Natural Progesterone Information Service
NPIS supplies women and their doctors with details on how to obtain natural progesterone, as well as providing info packs for the general public and health practitioners, books, tapes and videos relating to natural hormone health. For an order form and prescribing details, send an sae to NPIS, BCM Box 4315, London WC1N 3XX.

Mental Health Project
This is a voluntary action group, supported by ION, to inform the public about the role of nutrition in mental health, to promote the nutrition connection to health professionals, policy-makers and sufferers, and to provide resources to encourage more research and implementation of nutritional strategies to reduce mental suffering. If you'd like to help, call ION (see above) or send an sae.

DIRECTORY OF SUPPLEMENT MANUFACTURERS

Health Plus offer by mail order an extensive range of supplements including the *VV Pack – The Ultimate Vitamin and Mineral Programme*. They also supply *Get Up and Go*. Send for a free catalogue to: Health Plus Ltd, Dolphin House, 30 Lushington Road, Eastbourne, East Sussex BN21 4LL (tel: 01323 737374).

Healthcrafts produce an extensive range of supplements available from health food stores, pharmacies etc. One of the most popular products is *Prolonged Release Nutrition Mega Multis*. These are high-potency multivitamin and mineral tablets, specially designed to release their contents gradually to ensure an even supply of nutrients in sufficient amounts throughout the day. For information contact: Ferrosan Healthcare Ltd, Beaver House, York Close, Byfleet, Surrey KT14 7HN (tel: 01932 337700).

Higher Nature produce an extensive range of vitamin, mineral and herbal supplements. Their best multivitamin is the *Optimum Nutrition Formula*. They also supply *Get Up and Go* and *Essential Balance* oil blend. Free catalogue and newsletter from Higher Nature, Burwash Common, East Sussex TN19 7LX (tel: 01435 882880).

Larkhall/Green Farm produce two extensive ranges of vitamin and mineral supplements, available both through health food stores and mail order. Their best multivitamins are *Cantassium's Cantamega 2000* and *Natural Flow's Mega Multi*. Send for a free catalogue to: Larkhall/Green Farm, 225 Putney Bridge Road, London SW15 2PY (tel: 0181 874 1130).

Nature's Best produce an extensive range of vitamin and mineral supplements available by mail order. Their best multivitamin is *MultiGuard*. Write or telephone for a free 72-page colour catalogue to: Nature's Best Ltd, Freepost (Dept OH), PO Box 1, Tunbridge Wells, Kent TN2 3BR (tel: 01892 552118).

Solgar produce a wide range of supplements available from any good health food store. They include the award-winning *VM 2000* and *VM 75*. For stockists contact: Solgar Vitamins Ltd, Aldbury, Tring, Herts HP23 5PT (tel: 01442 890355).

INDEX